Student's

MATERNAL, NEONATAL, AND WOMEN'S HEALTH NURSING

Aileen MacLaren, CNM, MSN
Assistant Professor of Clinical Nursing
University of Miami

Springhouse Corporation
Springhouse, Pennsylvania

STAFF

Executive Director, Editorial
Stanley Loeb

Director of Trade and Textbooks
Minnie B. Rose, RN, BSN, MEd

Art Director
John Hubbard

Associate Acquisitions Editor
Betsy Steinmetz

Editor
Kathy Goldberg

Copy Editors
Mary Hohenhaus Hardy, Elizabeth Kiselev, Keith de Pinho

Designer
Julie Carleton Barlow

Manufacturing
Deborah Meiris (manager), T.A. Landis, Jennifer Suter

Production Coordinator
Caroline Lemoine

The clinical procedures described and recommended in this publication are based on currently accepted clinical theory and practice and on consultation with medical and nursing authorities. Nevertheless, they cannot be considered absolute and universal recommendations. Suggested activities and interventions must be considered in light of the client's clinical condition and, before administration of new or infrequently used drugs, in light of latest package-insert information. The authors and the publisher disclaim responsibility for any adverse effects resulting directly or indirectly from the suggested procedures, from any undetected errors, or from the reader's misunderstanding of the text.

ISBN 0-87434-360-7 RTMSAB 010391

CONTENTS

Advisory Board vi

Introduction vii

Unit One ◆ Nursing the Childbearing Family: History, Concepts, and Practice

1 ◆ **Family Nursing Care: History and Trends** 1
Sylvia A. McSkimming, RN, PhD; Carole Ann Kenner, RN,C, DNS

2 ◆ **Family Structure and Function** 3
Christine A. Grant, RN, PhD; Gale Robinson Smith, RN, PhD, CS

3 ◆ **Nursing Process and the Childbearing Family** 7
Gale Robinson Smith, RN, PhD, CS; Cynthia L. Armstrong, RN,C, MSN

4 ◆ **Nurse-Client Interaction** 10
Florencetta Gibson, RN, MSN, MEd

5 ◆ **Ethical and Legal Concerns in Family Care** 13
Sarah D. Cohn, CNM, MSN, JD

Unit Two ◆ Women's Health Care

6 ◆ **Reproductive Anatomy and Physiology** 16
Constance A. Bobik, RN, MSN

7 ◆ **Women's Health Promotion** 22
Linda Wheeler, CNM, MN, EdD

8 ◆ **Sexuality Concerns** 26
Catherine Ingram Fogel, RN,C, PhD; Barbara C. Rynerson, RN,C, MS

9 ◆ **Family Planning** 30
Lynne Hutnik Conrad, RN,C, MSN

10 ◆ **Fertility and Infertility** 35
Debra C. Davis, RN, DSN

11 ◆ **Genetics and Genetic Disorders** 39
Janet K. Williams, RN, PhD, CPNP

12 ◆ **Infectious Disorders** 43
Bonnie Mauger Graff, RN, MSN, CRNP

13 ◆ **Gynecologic Disorders** 47
Rosemary Theroux, RN,C, MS; Peggy Sherblom Matteson, RN,C, MS

14 ◆ **Violence Against Women** 51
Rosemary J. McKeighen, RN, PhD, CMFT, FAAN

15 ◆ **Women's Health-Compromising Behaviors** 55
Anne Myers Gudmundsen, RN, PhD

Unit Three: The Antepartal Period

16 ◆ **Conception and Fetal Development** 59
Leonard V. Crowley, MD; Susan M. Cohen, RN, DSN

17 ◆ **Physiologic Changes during Normal Pregnancy** 61
Bernadine Adams, RN, BSN, MN

18 ◆ **Psychosocial Changes during Normal Pregnancy** 65
Constance Sinclair, RN, MSN, CNM

19 ◆ **Care during the Normal Antepartal Period** 69
Christabel A. Kaitell, RN, BN, MPH, SCM

20 ◆ **Nutrition and Diet Counseling** 72
Ann Brodsky, MS, RD

21 ◆ **Family Preparation for Childbirth and Parenting** 75
Joan Engebretson, RN, MS; Harriett Linenberger, RN,C, MSN, ACCE-R

22 ◆ **High-Risk Antepartal Clients** 81
Patricia Anne Mynaugh, RN, PhD

23 ◆ **Antepartal Complications** 84
Catherine Dearman, RN, PhD

Unit Four: The Intrapartal Period

24 ◆ **Physiology of Labor and Childbirth** 88
Lynne Hutnik Conrad, RN,C, MSN

25 ◆ **Fetal Assessment** 93
Connie Marshall, RN, MSN

26 ◆ **Comfort Promotion during Labor and Childbirth** 97
Kathleen Convery Hanold, RN, MS

27 ◆ **The First Stage of Labor** 100
Aileen MacLaren, CNM, MSN

28 ◆ **The Second Stage of Labor** 104
Donna J. van Lier, CNM, PhD

29 ◆ **The Third and Fourth Stages of Labor** 106
Jan Weingrad Smith, CNM, MS, MPH

30 ◆ **Family Support during the Intrapartal Period** 109
Virginia H. Kemp, RN, PhD; Tommie P. Nelms, RN, PhD

31 ◆ **High-Risk Intrapartal Clients** 112
Aileen MacLaren, CNM, MSN; JoNell Efantis, RN, ARNP, MSN

32 ◆ **Special Obstetric Procedures** 115
Peggy J. Drapo, RN, PhD; Charlotte R. Patrick, RN, MS, MEd

33 ◆ Intrapartal Complications 118
Andrea O. Hollingsworth, RN, PhD

Unit Five: The Neonate

34 ◆ Neonatal Adaptation 121
Judy Wright Lott, ARNP, MSN

35 ◆ Neonatal Assessment 125
Darlene Nebel Cantu, RN,C, MSN: Laura Rodriguez Vaello, RN,C, MSN, NNP;
Carole Ann Kenner, RN,C, DNS

36 ◆ Care of the Normal Neonate 130
Carole Ann Kenner, RN,C, DNS

37 ◆ Infant Nutrition 132
Gail Blair Storr, RN, MN, MEd

38 ◆ High-Risk Neonates 136
Laurie Porter Gunderson, RN, PhD; Darlene Nebel Cantu, RN,C, MSN;
Laura Rodriguez Vaello, RN,C, MSN, NNP

39 ◆ Care of the Families of High-Risk Neonates 141
Ann E. Brueggemeyer, RN, MBA, MSN

40 ◆ Discharge Planning and Neonatal Care at Home 144
Brook Gumm, RN, MSN; Mary E. Lynch, RN, MS

Unit Six: The Postpartal Period

41 ◆ Physiology of the Postpartal Period 146
Deborah S. Davison, MSN, CRNP

42 ◆ Care during the Normal Postpartal Period 149
Harriett W. Ferguson, RN,C, EdD

43 ◆ Psychosocial Adaptation of the Postpartal Family 152
Sarah Elizabeth Whitaker, RN,C, MSN

44 ◆ Postpartal Complications 156
Paula Maisano Herndon, RN, MS

45 ◆ Maternal Care at Home 159
Annette Gupton, RN, MN

Answers for Chapters 1 through 45 162

ADVISORY BOARD

Kathleen G. Andreoli, RN, DSN, FAAN
Vice-President,
Nursing Affairs and The John L. and Helen Kellogg Dean,
College of Nursing,
Rush-Presbyterian–St. Luke's Medical Center/Rush University,
Chicago

Marie Scott Brown, RN, PhD
Pediatric Nurse Practitioner,
Professor of Family Nursing, School of Nursing,
Oregon Health Science University,
Portland

Kathleen Dracup, RN, DNSc, FAAN
Professor, School of Nursing,
University of California,
Los Angeles

Elizabeth Grossman, RN, EdD, FAAN
Professor of Nursing,
Indiana University School of Nursing,
Indianapolis

Evelyn R. Hayes, RN, PhD
Associate Professor, College of Nursing,
University of Delaware,
Newark

Mary D. Naylor, RN, PhD, FAAN
Associate Dean and Director of Undergraduate Studies,
School of Nursing, University of Pennsylvania,
Philadelphia

INTRODUCTION

The student who would achieve excellence in maternal, neonatal, and women's health nursing must combine sound theoretical knowledge with compassionate clinical practice. This means developing a rich knowledge base and mastering skills that are appropriate to each specific clinical setting.

Student's Activities Book reviews facts and skills application and challenges the student in applying theory to practice. The activities accompany and complement the Cohen, Kenner, and Hollingsworth textbook, *Maternal, Neonatal, and Women's Health Nursing*. Because the answers to the activities derive directly from procedures and explanations in the textbook, the student must be familiar with the information there to answer the questions correctly.

Student's Activities Book uses various strategies to help the student meet the learning objectives for each textbook chapter, understand the concepts discussed, and apply these concepts to clinical situations. Each chapter presents an overview of key concepts and then offers clinical simulations and various types of activities. Based on brief case studies, the clinical simulations integrate major concepts from the text chapter and relate these concepts to clinical practice. Multiple-choice questions challenge the student to select correctly from among related information; study questions call for explanations of appropriate interventions; true-or-false statements test recall and command of facts; matching exercises call for pairing related elements; fill-in-the-blank statements test understanding of information in specific contexts; anatomic illustrations for labeling check knowledge of precise details; and values clarification exercises prompt self-examination. This rich variety of activities should stimulate and direct thinking, evaluation of one's knowledge base, and any necessary additional study. Answers provide details and refer to appropriate textbook pages so that the student can review material should clarification and reinforcement be needed.

◆ CHAPTER 1 ◆

FAMILY NURSING CARE: HISTORY AND TRENDS

CHAPTER OVERVIEW

Chapter 1 explores basic concepts regarding the family, discusses the role of family nursing care, and describes significant historical events that have affected nursing and women. It investigates recent social and economic trends, tracing their relationship to women's changing roles and the emergence of a consumer-oriented approach to health care. The chapter surveys the expanding and varied roles of advanced nursing practice for the childbearing family and highlights the historical development of nurse-midwifery as an example of the evolution of nurse-specialist roles within family-centered health care. It discusses trends in nursing research and current research priorities in parent and child health.

STUDENT ACTIVITIES

To test your familiarity with the information in this chapter, complete the following activities.

Multiple choice

1. In the mid-1800s, the Industrial Revolution led to significant changes in family structure and roles. Which of the following statements describes a specific effect of the Industrial Revolution on the family?
(a) Families became less self-sufficient.
(b) Women had considerable opportunities for advanced education.
(c) The philosophy of humanism emerged, promoting the concept of the individual's dignity, worth, and capacity for self-realization.
(d) Family functions became more cohesive.

2. The use of diagnosis-related groups (DRGs) to reimburse health care facilities for client care has:
(a) played a minor role in the economics of health care
(b) prompted health care facilities to discharge clients as early as possible
(c) eliminated the need for professional standards review organizations
(d) reduced the demand for home health care services

Study questions

3. Regardless of its composition, the family fulfills certain basic functions for its members. Describe the affective, socialization and social placement, reproductive, economic, and health functions of the family.

4. How did the Industrial Revolution affect health care and family nursing?

5. Which four major concepts of nursing did Florence Nightingale propose, and how have these concepts affected the practice of family nursing today?

6. What was the Goldmark Report, and how did it influence the development of nursing education?

7. Name four recent social trends that have had a significant impact on women and their families.

8. Many women in today's work force are mothers. What are some important issues facing these women that influence family nursing care?

9. Which two current social trends have stimulated women to participate more actively in their own health care?

10. Name five cost-containment measures adopted by the health care industry that have resulted in significant changes in client reimbursement, health care delivery, and facility operation.

11. Why does Canada have a lower infant mortality rate than the United States, despite spending less of its gross national product on health care?

12. What are the drawbacks of Canada's National Health Program, compared with the U.S. health care system?

13. Today's nurse may assume many roles in family care. Give an example of how a maternal, neonatal, or women's health care nurse can fulfill the following roles: advocate, educator, change agent, and nurse-researcher.

14. In which two ways can nurse-researchers contribute to nursing care of women and their families?

15. Describe the differences in clinical focus for a certified nurse-midwife, a family nurse practitioner, and a neonatal nurse practitioner.

Fill in the blank

16. The transformation of the United States from an industrial society to an ____________ society means that the nurse must think critically and be technically competent in order to assimilate new information rapidly and apply it appropriately.

17. The transition to a highly technological society requires high touch, demonstrated in nursing through ____________ and ____________.

◆ CHAPTER 2 ◆

FAMILY STRUCTURE AND FUNCTION

CHAPTER OVERVIEW

Families form the foundation of our society. Each family is a discrete unit of individuals who share an emotional involvement and live in proximity. Chapter 2 discusses the types of families that the nurse may encounter, explores the functions of the family, and examines typical roles and patterns of relationships within families. To help the nurse work more effectively with the childbearing family, the chapter identifies coping mechanisms that help maintain family functioning during crises.

STUDENT ACTIVITIES

To test your familiarity with the information in this chapter, complete the following activities.

Clinical simulations

1. Anne Foster, age 42, delivered her son Jonathan 6 weeks ago. When conducting the postpartal family assessment, the nurse learns that Anne and her husband, Jerry, have been married for 8 years and that their family has experienced many changes during the past year. Jerry, who has a successful but demanding law practice, turned 50. Meagan, their older child, is nearly age 4 and began preschool recently. Anne has decided to resign from her job as a television producer to stay home and raise her children full time. Both of the children's grandmothers live in distant cities and cannot help with child care. Each paragraph below presents an interpretation of the Foster family based on one of the following family theories: developmental theory, interactional theory, social exchange theory, structural-functional theory, or systems theory. Identify the theory expressed in each paragraph.
(a) The Fosters are a nuclear family with traditional values that holds to the conservative belief that child rearing is the sole responsibility of the immediate family, with the mother as primary caregiver.
(b) The relationship between Anne and Jerry influences individual family members. The couple's loving relationship and contentment with their children affect their interactions with each other. Anne's early postpartal fatigue had a dramatic impact on Jerry and consequently altered their interactions with Meagan and Jonathan.
(c) Before Jonathan was born, Anne had planned to return to her job part time as a television producer. However, the unanticipated demands of raising a second child caused stress between her and Jerry as they tried to coordinate their child-care responsibilities.

After considering her options and their ramifications, Anne decided to resign from her job. Her decision minimized the costs to her marriage and family life and maximized the rewards.
(d) Jonathan's birth created a subsystem that changed the original system formed by Anne, Jerry, and Meagan. Anne's ability to take on various roles—wife, mother, and career woman—indicates open family boundaries, promoting adaptation to the birth of a second child.
(e) The Foster family is in stage 3 of their family life cycle. Meagan is beginning preschool and slowly shifting from dependence to self-reliance as she learns proper social behavior away from home.

2. Judy Bevis learns she is pregnant during her final exams at law school. After a brief discussion, she and her fiance, Scott, decide to get married in a civil ceremony 2 months before their scheduled church wedding. Within 3 weeks, Judy and Scott have moved into a new apartment and made plans for Judy's graduation from law school. Judy then has a miscarriage. What are some factors Judy's nurse should assess to anticipate how well she and Scott will respond to this family crisis? Are Judy and Scott experiencing a maturational crisis or situational crisis? Explain your answer.

3. Sylvia Smith, age 24, has a 4-year-old son and an 18-month-old daughter. Recently, her husband left the family, resulting in financial problems that forced Sylvia and her children to move into a cramped one-bedroom apartment. What are some consequences of single parenthood that the nurse should anticipate for Sylvia?

Study questions

4. Briefly define family theory.

5. Identify each of the family developmental stages described below, as defined by Duvall:
(a) Besides adjusting to each child's life-style choices, parents establish new ties and renegotiate their marital relationship as their children depart.
(b) Changes in activities and declining health and energy alter family configurations.
(c) Parents are faced with their child's growing autonomy and independence while they begin to revive their own personal interests and issues.
(d) The partners clarify their marital roles and expectations and make decisions about parenthood.
(e) The parents and child adjust to new boundaries between them as the child shifts slowly from dependence to self-reliance and learns proper social behavior through parental reinforcement.
(f) The last child leaves the home; the partners may be unhappy about their home lives or careers and anxious about aging and death.
(g) The first child is integrated into the family unit, leading to the most significant change in a marriage; the couple must adapt to their new roles and to the responsibilities of parenting.
(h) The child learns from people outside the family and develops a self-identity; parents adjust to peer influences on their child.

6. Identify and define three variations on the contemporary nuclear family.

7. For each of the situations described below, identify the type of family role conflict that is occurring.
(a) Role expectations differ among family members.
(b) A family member assumes too many roles and, as a result, cannot fulfill the expectations of each role.
(c) A family member's internal values differ from those required to fulfill role responsibilities.

8. When helping a client cope with a crisis, the nurse can provide different types of social support, depending on the client's special needs. Identify and describe the three types of social support.

Fill in the blank

9. The __________ family theory proposes that families seek to maintain a stable societal structure by organizing around traditional sex-based role relationships and conservative beliefs.

10. By emphasizing relationships, the __________ family theory facilitates identification of potential problems between family members.

11. The reciprocal relationship between partners and the interplay of individual motives, perceptions, and behaviors is the central tenet of the __________ family theory.

Matching terms and definitions

12. The examples provided in the left column describe various functions that family members typically carry out by adopting recurrent behavior patterns, or roles. Match each function with the corresponding role shown in the right column.

(1) person who assumes responsibility for each family member's accountability by assigning family tasks and delegating responsibilities to achieve family goals	(a) provider
(2) person who keeps track of and celebrates birthdays, anniversaries, holidays, and family customs	(b) nurturer
(3) person who continually explores and clarifies the family's belief system, establishing standards and enforcing acceptable behavior	(c) decision maker

(4) person who monitors the personal well-being of family members by suggesting standards for diet, hygiene, grooming, and exercise and by establishing responses to illness and health	(d) problem solver
(5) primary person who offers love, support, care, reassurance, and comfort to maintain or increase each family member's personal development	(e) tradition setter
(6) person who ensures that the family has food, clothing, shelter, and money	(f) value setter
(7) health supervisor	(g) health supervisor

◆ CHAPTER 3 ◆

NURSING PROCESS AND THE CHILDBEARING FAMILY

CHAPTER OVERVIEW

Nursing care of the childbearing family has grown increasingly complex over the past 50 years as family structures and functions have changed. Contemporary nursing has developed an organized framework, called the nursing process, to provide comprehensive care that addresses families' wide-ranging health needs. Providing a system for making nursing decisions, the nursing process steps include assessment, nursing diagnosis, planning, implementation, and evaluation. Chapter 3 examines each of these steps, showing how the nurse uses them to help ensure high-quality, family-centered nursing care and to develop effective strategies for meeting current or potential health care needs of childbearing or child-rearing families. It also explains how to incorporate thorough documentation into nursing care for these families.

STUDENT ACTIVITIES

To test your familiarity with the information in this chapter, complete the following activities.

Clinical simulations

1. Wanda Mallaro, age 25, recently moved to the United States from the Philippines. Two months ago—just days after she found out she was pregnant—her husband died in a car accident. Now, 15 weeks into her pregnancy, she makes her first prenatal visit to the clinic, accompanied by her mother and 3-year-old son. Which three broad categories of family differences should the nurse who addresses Wanda investigate? Which relevant data should the nurse collect?

2. During the assessment, the nurse discovers that Wanda has poor coping skills. Which potential consequence of poor coping should the nurse keep in mind while formulating her plan of care?

3. When providing nursing care for Wanda and her family, how can the nurse avoid an ethnocentric approach in which vital information is overlooked?

4. Identify three nursing diagnoses that are appropriate for Wanda and her family during this pregnancy.

Study questions

5. After collecting a health history specific to a prenatal client's pregnancy concerns, the nurse should explore which other areas of in-

fluence during a thorough assessment of the client and her adaptation to pregnancy?

6. Identify the three basic steps in the planning phase of the nursing process.

7. What are the benefits of client involvement in goal setting?

8. When does the implementation phase of the nursing process begin and end?

9. List the characteristics of an effective goal statement.

10. Identify the segments of a complete nursing diagnosis.

11. What are the four types of skills the nurse needs to implement nursing interventions successfully?

12. Name the three major functions of documentation of nursing care.

13. Although regulations regarding the minimal frequency of documentation may differ among states and institutions, which guidelines must the nurse always follow when documenting client care?

Fill in the blank

14. When performing the assessment, gather __________ data directly from the client or family members, and collect __________ data by conducting a physical examination or using other medical or nursing sources.

15. To convey interest and encourage the client to talk during the health history interview, be sure to use effective body language, such as leaning forward, nodding periodically, and __________.

16. Although __________ is considered the last step of the nursing process, it actually occurs throughout all the steps, especially during __________ when the nurse reassesses the effectiveness of interventions.

17. The basis for formulating an individualized, effective nursing care plan is the __________, which provides a common language to convey the necessary nursing management.

Matching terms and definitions

18. To gain confidence when using the nursing process, the nurse should be familiar with each step as well as its purpose. Match each description in the left column with the corresponding nursing pro-

cess step shown in the right column. Then rearrange the steps in their proper sequence.

(1) nursing actions that carry out the interventions described in the care plan to achieve the established goals	(a) planning
(2) determination of how successfully the goals of the care plan have been met	(b) nursing diagnosis
(3) setting and prioritizing of goals for each nursing diagnosis, formulation of interventions to achieve the goals, and development of a nursing care plan	(c) assessment
(4) descriptive statement identifying actual or potential client health problem that can be resolved or diminished by nursing care	(d) evaluation
(5) systematic collection of information about the client's health status	(e) implementation

Proper sequence of steps:

Step 1: ____________

Step 2: ____________

Step 3: ____________

Step 4: ____________

Step 5: ____________

◆ CHAPTER 4 ◆

NURSE-CLIENT INTERACTION

CHAPTER OVERVIEW

Developing an effective ongoing relationship with the client and family is an important part of nursing care for obstetric, gynecologic, and neonatal clients. During nurse-client interaction, the nurse must determine any special client health care needs or desires, establish specific health care goals, and provide the particular type of nursing care required. Chapter 4 describes the five characteristic phases of nurse-client interaction. It explains how the nurse initiates and directs these phases and emphasizes the importance of active client participation to ensure successful interaction. The chapter also examines the key psychosocial nursing skills needed to achieve optimal client outcomes—communicating, teaching, and motivating.

STUDENT ACTIVITIES

To test your familiarity with the information in this chapter, complete the following activities.

Clinical simulations

1. Francine Morgan, a public health nurse, is planning a home visit to Sally Weitzman, a 26-year-old client who is 26 weeks' pregnant. Sally will be discharged from the health care facility today after stabilization for preterm labor. Which steps should Francine take to prepare for the initial home visit?

2. During the initial visit to Sally's home, which steps should Francine take to establish rapport with Sally and initiate nurse-client interaction?

3. Which general tasks should Francine accomplish during the consolidation and growth phase of her interaction with Sally?

4. Although Francine prepared Sally for termination of the nurse-client interaction during initiation and has reminded her periodically that termination is a planned phase, Sally expresses feelings of sadness and abandonment as termination approaches. How should Francine deal with Sally's feelings?

5. At a family planning clinic, Pearl Green, a 17-year-old pregnant client, complains of "terrible sores down there." After she is diagnosed with herpes genitalis, she asks how she could have gotten this disease. Of the following statements, which represents the most appropriate response to Pearl's question? State the rationale for your answer.
   (a) "Many sexually active teenagers get this kind of problem when

they're not careful, just like you."
(b) "Why do you think this happened to you now?"
(c) "Adolescents have no business being sexually active. This was inevitable."
(d) "I see this is making you worried and uncomfortable. What do you know about this disease?"

6. To convey empathy during Pearl's exit interview, the nurse slides the chair closer to Pearl's and puts a hand on her shoulder. Pearl becomes uncomfortable and seems reluctant to answer further questions about her sexual history. What is the probable cause of her sudden discomfort, and which steps should the nurse take to put her at ease?

7. To teach Pearl effectively, the nurse must address learning characteristics specific to her age group. What are some characteristics the nurse must keep in mind when formulating a teaching strategy for Pearl?

8. Bettina Bird, age 38, had her first child by cesarean delivery 3 days ago. Entering Bettina's room for a teaching session on breast-feeding, the nurse sees that Bettina has been crying. She complains that her breasts feel warm and hard, that her nipples are tender, and that she experiences "excruciating" pain when her son attempts to breast-feed. After determining that Bettina is experiencing normal breast engorgement, the nurse should consider which of the following as the highest priority for Bettina's breast-feeding education? Explain your answer.
(a) determining her knowledge level about breast-feeding (such as from books and her friends' experiences)
(b) evaluating her interest in learning about breast-feeding and her commitment to this feeding method
(c) overcoming her discomfort from breast engorgement and identifying any other obstacles to learning before proceeding with the session
(d) determining her learning style

9. Lynne, a primigravid client age 20 who is 25 weeks pregnant, has been diagnosed with iron-deficiency anemia. How can the nurse at the prenatal clinic that Lynne attends foster her self-care to improve her nutrition during pregnancy?

Study questions

10. What is the major disadvantage of individual client teaching?

11. Identify at least three guidelines for successful team teaching.

12. Name and describe the learning styles identified by Kolb.

Fill in the blank

13. The most important measure of teaching effectiveness is how much the client __________ .

14. __________ allows the nurse to care for and motivate the client by recognizing and viewing experiences from the client's perspective in a sensitive yet professional manner.

Matching terms and definitions

15. Match each definition in the left column with the corresponding glossary term in the right column.

(1) process in which the nurse and client agree on goals and anticipated outcomes before teaching begins	(a) active listening
(2) failure to act in accordance with wishes, requests, demands, or requirements	(b) body language
(3) interaction that focuses on attaining client goals rather than on the mutual pleasure received from social communication	(c) contract learning
(4) person whose skill, aptitude, or experience eases task performance	(d) facilitator
(5) close evaluation of body language and voice inflection to supplement verbal communication	(e) learning style
(6) teaching strategy in which the nurse asks nonthreatening follow-up questions after each teaching session	(f) noncompliance
(7) client's preferred way of absorbing or recalling information; for example, memorization, observation, interaction, and experimentation	(g) operant conditioning
(8) repeated rewards that encourage specific behaviors	(h) programmed learning
(9) nonverbal signals, such as facial expression, gestures, and body position	(i) self-care
(10) active and assertive participation in attaining one's health care goals	(j) therapeutic communication

◆ CHAPTER 5 ◆

ETHICAL AND LEGAL CONCERNS IN FAMILY CARE

CHAPTER OVERVIEW

The nurse caring for maternal and neonatal clients may confront ethical dilemmas daily. Dealing confidently with such dilemmas and protecting against unnecessary liability require a solid grounding in the ethical and legal principles involved. Chapter 5 explores the principles that govern ethical decision making and discusses how ethics relates to professional nursing standards and to the law. It presents strategies the nurse can use to minimize legal risks and provides examples of the ethical and legal dilemmas that arise in maternal, neonatal, and women's health care.

STUDENT ACTIVITIES

To test your familiarity with the information in this chapter, complete the following activities.

Clinical simulations

1. Rosalie Garcia, a recently married, 20-year-old client, is 8 weeks pregnant. During the health history interview, she confides hesitantly that she has had two uncomplicated abortions. However, she does not want her husband to know about them and asks the nurse not to document them on her medical record. Her request places the nurse in an ethical bind, because her wishes conflict with the nurse's responsibility to document a complete health history. Also, the nurse believes in total honesty and communication within marriage. How should the nurse decide on a course of action?

2. Adeline Younger has just left her physician's office after giving informed consent for a sterilization procedure. In the hall, she takes the nurse aside and asks if the incision will "look as big and hurt as much as a cesarean section." From this question, the nurse suspects that Mrs. Younger is confused about or lacks a complete understanding of the procedure. What is the nurses' legal responsibility in this case, and what, if any, action should the nurse take?

Study questions

3. List the three professional purposes of a nurse practice act.

4. How does the model proposed by Bunting and Webb help the nurse make an ethical decision? Describe this model.

5. Identify the four elements of malpractice liability that the plaintiff must prove to win a malpractice lawsuit against a nurse.

6. Why are student nurses subject to a charge of negligence even when under the supervision of a graduate nurse?

7. Although a nurse who makes an error is liable personally and professionally, the employer also is responsible. Which principle of law applies here, and what are the legal consequences of this principle?

8. Mrs. Martinez is in the last trimester of her fourth pregnancy. She and her husband have decided on a tubal ligation for contraception after their child is born and determined to be healthy. To ensure informed consent, what in formation should the physician provide to Mrs. Martinez and her husband about the sterilization?

9. List the three main goals of risk management.

True or false

10. The American Nurses' Association Code for Nurses provides ethical standards of conduct and guidelines for all aspects of nursing practice.
❑ True ❑ False

11. Nurse practice acts typically prohibit specific nursing functions that might compromise professional standards.
❑ True ❑ False

12. Although many laws are based on ethical principles, the nurse usually cannot depend on laws to define personal ethical standards.
❑ True ❑ False

13. In a few select cases, a specific law can be ignored with impunity, such as when an individual strongly believes that the law is ethically wrong.
❑ True ❑ False

14. Incident reports that are written clearly and concisely immediately after an occurrence may substitute for medical record documentation during legal proceedings.
❑ True ❑ False

15. The principles of malpractice or professional liability are different for nurses than for physicians and other health care professionals.
❑ True ❑ False

16. If a physician does not respond to a serious problem (such as fetal distress), the nurse is obligated legally to notify a supervisor, who must arrange appropriate emergency care for the client.
❑ True ❑ False

17. When documenting nursing care, the nurse may erase an error as long as the correction is legible and initialed.
❑ True ❑ False

Fill in the blank

18. To make an ethical decision, the nurse must learn how to ____________, identify the ethical dimensions of nursing practice, and relate ethical decisions to clinical practice.

19. One of the most difficult aspects of ethics in nursing involves the principle of ____________, which holds that the client's ethical decisions take precedence over the nurse's convictions.

20. Unlike the deontological approach to ethics, which bases ethical principles on ____________, the teleological approach bases ethical principles on ____________.

21. The ____________ is a primary legal resource for nursing that governs the functions of the profession for each state.

Matching terms and definitions

22. Match each definition in the left column with the corresponding glossary term in the right column.

(1) lawsuit addressing the rights and duties of private persons	(a) negligence
(2) person against whom a lawsuit is brought	(b) malpractice
(3) legal rule in which a client is entitled to receive certain information about a proposed course of treatment or surgery	(c) defendant
(4) obligation to pay monetary damages in a civil action	(d) civil action
(5) form of negligence action brought against professionals that alleges failure to meet applicable standards, thus causing harm	(e) plaintiff
(6) failure to act as a reasonable person given similar training, experience, and circumstances would act	(f) informed consent
(7) person who initiates a lawsuit	(g) liability

◆ CHAPTER 6 ◆

REPRODUCTIVE ANATOMY AND PHYSIOLOGY

CHAPTER OVERVIEW

The nurse who provides family-centered care for women and their partners during the childbearing years must possess an in-depth knowledge of the anatomy and physiology of the reproductive system. Chapter 6 provides a detailed discussion of the structures and functions of the female and male reproductive systems, providing the knowledge base necessary to develop a plan of care. It describes the female external and internal genitalia, discusses the breasts, and illustrates pelvic structure and pelvic floor musculature. It explains how hormones affect the development of the female reproductive system and discusses the relationship between the ovarian and endometrial cycles within the menstrual cycle. Then the chapter focuses on the anatomy and physiology of the male reproductive system, discussing male reproductive structures and spermatogenesis.

STUDENT ACTIVITIES

To test your familiarity with the information in this chapter, complete the following activities.

Study questions

1. What are the four basic pelvic types?

2. Describe the four stages of spermatogenesis.

3. For each description below, identify the corresponding female reproductive organ or structure.
   (a) almond-shaped organ located on either side of the uterus that produces mature ova
   (b) highly elastic muscular tube situated between the bladder and rectum along the midline of the body
   (c) hoodlike covering situated where the upper lamellae of the labia join
   (d) hollow, pear-shaped organ with thick, muscular walls located behind the symphysis pubis and bladder
   (e) complex structure between the lower vagina and the anal canal made up of muscles, fascia, blood vessels, nerves, and lymphatics
   (f) long, narrow structures that transport ova between the ovaries and uterus
   (g) highly vascular and innervated erectile tissue with marked sexual sensitivity
   (h) two small vulvovaginal structures, located deep in the perineal structure, that open into the lateral margins of the vaginal orifice

4. Describe the functions of the (a) uterosacral, (b) cardinal, (c) ovarian, (d) round, and (e) broad uterine ligaments.

5. What are the three functions of the perineal muscles?

6. Name the simultaneous cycles that make up the menstrual cycle.

7. Which hormone increases the sex drive in females and stimulates spermatogenesis in males?

8. Which endocrine gland produces the gonadotropic hormones, follicle-stimulating hormone (FSH), luteinizing hormone (LH), and prolactin?

Fill in the blank

9. The three tissue layers that make up the uterine corpus are called the ___________, ___________, and ___________.

10. The ___________ muscles originate at the ischial tuberosities and enter the perineum to form the urethral and vaginal sphincters.

11. The onset of cyclical menstrual periods is called ___________.

12. ___________ is the time when female reproductive ability ceases.

13. Hormonal production decreases and menses become irregular during the transition period known as the ___________.

14. Two clinical signs of ovulation are the abdominal pain in the ovarian region known as ___________ and the elastic cervical mucus discharge known as ___________.

15. During the endometrial cycle, the ___________ phase occurs as estrogen increases and the endometrial lining thickens before ovulation.

16. The secretory phase of the endometrial cycle begins after ovulation, when ___________ is released by the corpus luteum.

17. The menstrual phase of the endometrial cycle begins on the ___________ day of menses and lasts approximately ___________ days.

18. The hormones responsible for growth of the ovarian follicle are ___________ and ___________ .

19. The cervix is composed of ___________, ___________, and ___________.

Matching terms and definitions

20. Match each breast structure listed in the left column with the corresponding function in the right column.

(1) tiny, saclike duct terminals that secrete milk	(a) acini cells
(2) pigmented erectile tissue that responds to cold, friction, or stimulation	(b) Cooper's ligaments
(3) structures that store milk during lactation	(c) lobes
(4) sebaceous glands found on the areolar surface	(d) nipples
(5) structures containing the acini	(e) Montgomery's tubercles
(6) fibrous supportive structures of the breast	(f) ampullae (lactiferous ducts and sinuses)
(7) multiple openings in the nipple surface	(g) lactiferous ducts

Identification of anatomic structures

21. External female genitalia. In the illustration below, identify each structure next to the corresponding letter.

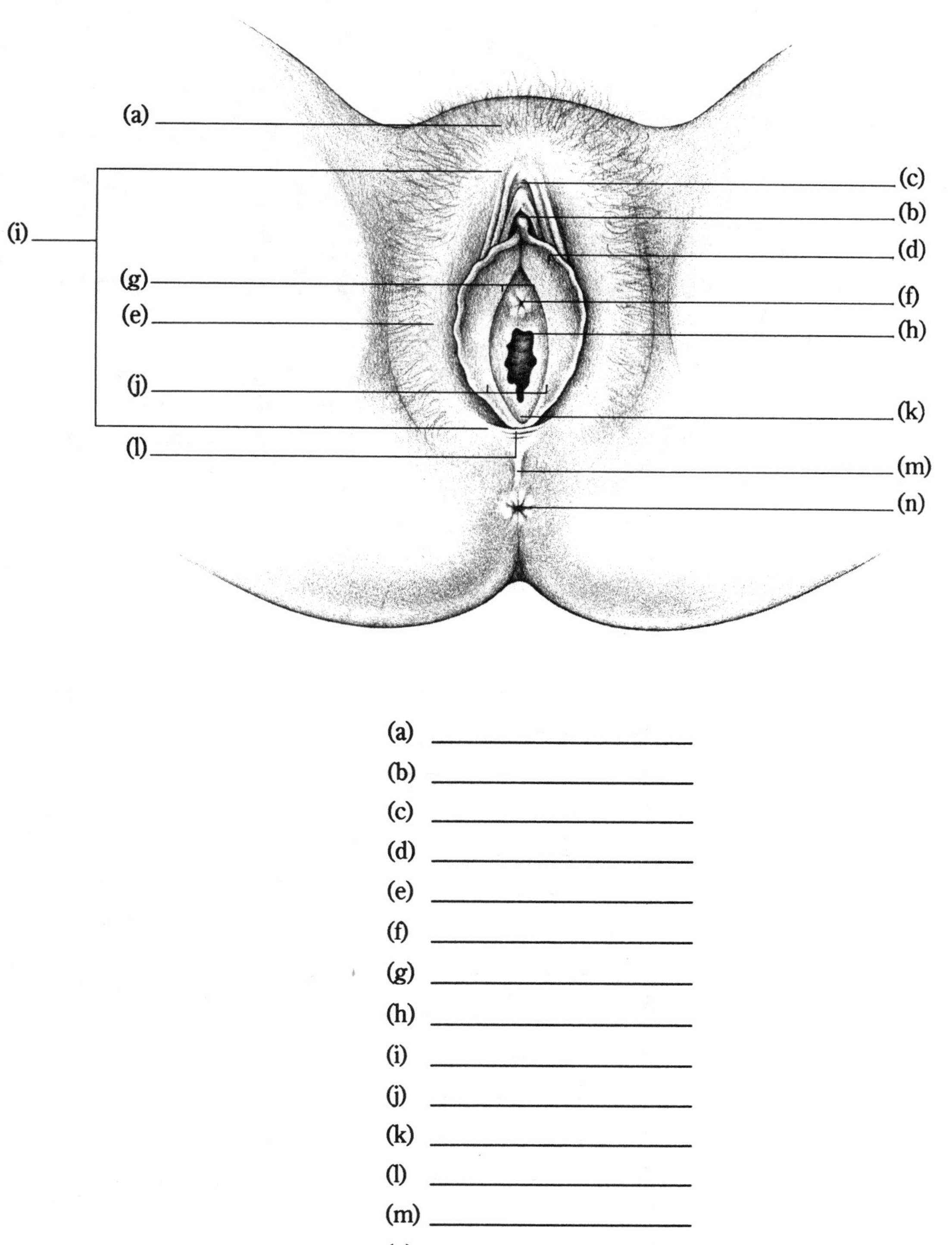

(a) ______________________

(b) ______________________

(c) ______________________

(d) ______________________

(e) ______________________

(f) ______________________

(g) ______________________

(h) ______________________

(i) ______________________

(j) ______________________

(k) ______________________

(l) ______________________

(m) ______________________

(n) ______________________

22. Internal female genitalia. In the illustration below, identify each structure next to the corresponding letter.

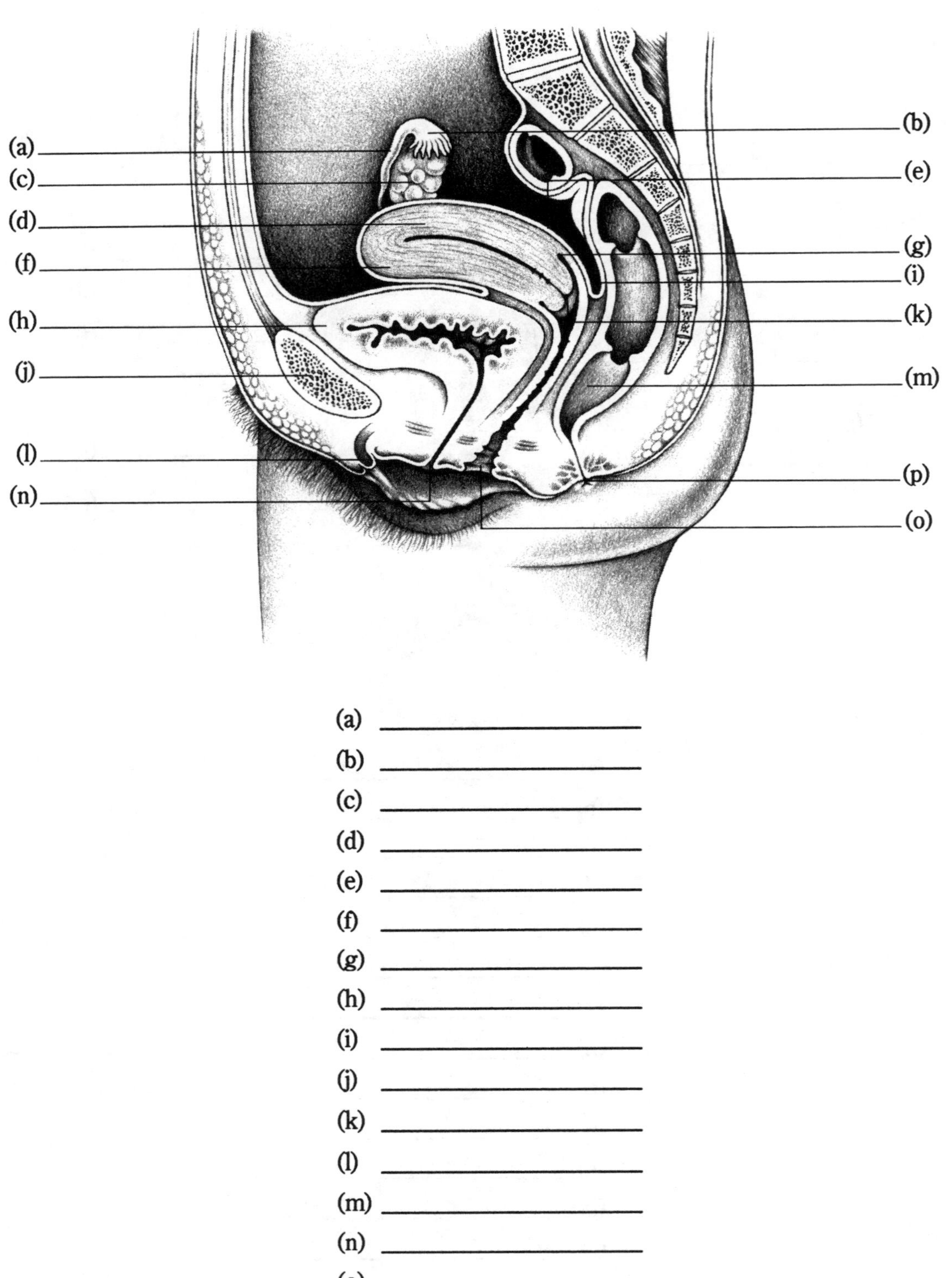

(a) ______________________

(b) ______________________

(c) ______________________

(d) ______________________

(e) ______________________

(f) ______________________

(g) ______________________

(h) ______________________

(i) ______________________

(j) ______________________

(k) ______________________

(l) ______________________

(m) ______________________

(n) ______________________

(o) ______________________

(p) ______________________

23. Internal male genitalia. In the illustration below, identify each structure next to the corresponding letter.

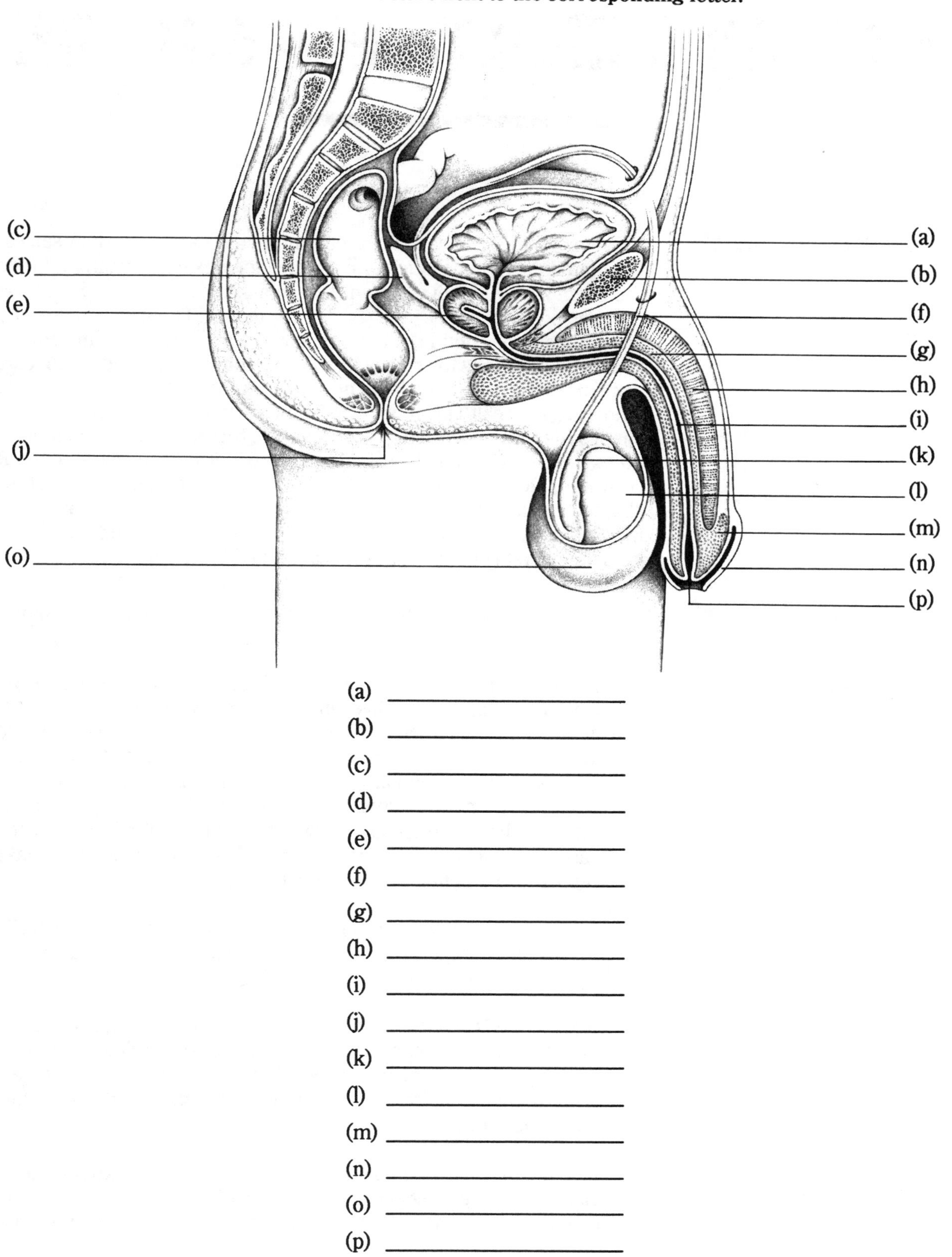

(a) ____________________

(b) ____________________

(c) ____________________

(d) ____________________

(e) ____________________

(f) ____________________

(g) ____________________

(h) ____________________

(i) ____________________

(j) ____________________

(k) ____________________

(l) ____________________

(m) ____________________

(n) ____________________

(o) ____________________

(p) ____________________

◆ CHAPTER 7 ◆

WOMEN'S HEALTH PROMOTION

CHAPTER OVERVIEW

Women are the primary consumers of health care—for themselves and their families. Gynecologic nursing care includes not only an evaluation of the client's reproductive system but an assessment of her health habits and her perceptions of her health care needs. Thus, such care encompasses health promotion, screening, counseling, advocacy, and education. Chapter 7 examines the role of health promotion in holistic health care for women, exploring gynecologic needs across the life span. It explains how to investigate health promotion and protection behaviors when taking the client's history, describes how to conduct the physical examination, and notes the developmental variations to consider during assessment. After reviewing the diagnostic tests used to evaluate gynecologic status, the chapter explains how to develop and implement the care plan, detailing health promotion activities to incorporate into client teaching. It highlights guidelines that enhance communication and teaching.

STUDENT ACTIVITIES

To test your familiarity with the information in this chapter, complete the following activities.

Clinical simulations

1. Esther Thompson is a 42-year-old client with five children. Originally from Jamaica, she now lives in the inner city region of a large urban area. As a single unemployed mother raising her last two children, ages 15 and 17, she relies on government assistance for health care. Ms. Thompson has avoided regular yearly examinations. Now, however, after experiencing menstrual irregularities for several months, she reluctantly visits the public health clinic to seek care. What factors may have deterred Ms. Thompson from making regular visits to health care providers?

2. When caring for Ms. Thompson—or for any perimenopausal client from a different cultural background—which considerations should the nurse keep in mind?

3. Stacey, age 15, comes to the health center because her mother wants her to obtain birth control information. However, Stacey's major concern is her menstruation, which began 6 months ago; she asks if her period is "normal." What information should the nurse give Stacey about the normal menstrual cycle?

4. Stacey reports that she and her boyfriend are not sexually active because Stacey feels she is not ready for this. Nonetheless, the nurse can use this visit to teach Stacey about contraception and disease

prevention. What are some teaching topics that might be appropriate for her at this time?

5. Joan, a 25-year-old accountant, has not had a gynecologic examination since college. During the health history interview, the nurse routinely questions her about her sexual preferences. Hesitantly, Joan divulges that she has been in a lesbian relationship for 3 years. What is the probable reason why Joan, like many of her homosexual peers, has avoided regular reproductive health care and hesitated to disclose her sexual orientation?

6. Patty Breeze, a 21-year-old client who recently relocated from another state, calls to schedule an annual gynecologic appointment. How can the nurse help Patty prepare for this visit?

7. Freda Gunter, age 52, has two adult children and three grandchildren. On her routine annual gynecologic examination, findings indicate the normal processes of aging and menopause. However, the physician is concerned about Mrs. Gunter's risk for osteoporosis because she has a family history of osteoporosis, is thin and petite (5′3″ tall, 115 lb), and reports that she gets little exercise. Also, her fair complexion, dry skin, and atrophic vaginitis signal menopausal changes. The nurse makes a nursing diagnosis of ***potential for injury related to decreased bone mass.***

After discussing hormone replacement therapy with her physician, Mrs. Gunter decides against this treatment. Based on the nursing diagnosis and Mrs. Gunter's unwillingness to begin hormone replacement therapy, describe appropriate nursing goals, implementation, and evaluation for her.

Study questions

8. List some typical reasons why pediatric clients visit a gynecologist.

9. What are the benefits of an educational pelvic examination?

10. Describe how the nurse can help avoid causing genital trauma when withdrawing a speculum during a pelvic examination.

11. List at least five recommendations that can help the nurse provide appropriate care for a lesbian client.

12. To assess the client's health promotion and protection behaviors, the nurse should investigate which specific topics?

13. List some topics the nurse should include when assessing a client's roles and relationships.

14. Breast examination includes both inspection and palpation. Which features should the nurse note when inspecting the breasts? What is the proper procedure for breast palpation?

15. List some breast palpation findings that indicate an abnormality.

16. During client teaching about breast self-examination (BSE), the nurse should instruct the client to perform BSE how often and at what point in the menstrual cycle?

17. What are normal expected findings of bimanual palpation during the pelvic examination?

18. Identify the health promotion concerns of adolescent women, childbearing women, perimenopausal women, and elderly women.

True or false

19. From the onset of menarche, regular menstrual cycles are established that last consistently from 3 to 7 days and repeat every 30 days.
❑ True ❑ False

20. Pregnancy is a possible cause of amenorrhea in childbearing clients.
❑ True ❑ False

21. Questioning a client about a miscarriage, stillbirth, or other perinatal loss is inappropriate because it invades the client's privacy.
❑ True ❑ False

22. Removal of the ovaries (oophorectomy) does not alter the menstrual cycle except when it is accompanied by a hysterectomy.
❑ True ❑ False

Matching related elements

23. The physician may order various laboratory tests for a gynecologic client. Match each test purpose in the left column with the corresponding test in the right column.

(1) screens for hyperlipidemia, which commonly occurs after menopause and increases a woman's risk for heart disease	(a) wet smear
(2) evaluates for glycosuria, proteinuria, and bacterial infection	(b) cervical cultures
(3) may reveal *Neisseria gonorrhoeae* or *Chlamydia trachomatis* infection	(c) HIV antibody test
(4) detects antibodies to the virus causing acquired immunodeficiency syndrome (AIDS)	(d) complete blood count
(5) identifies preinvasive and invasive cervical cancer	(e) Papanicolaou test
(6) screens for syphilis	(f) fecal occult blood test or Hematest
(7) screens for anemia and identifies infection that may stem from a sexually transmitted disease	(g) urinalysis

(8) may detect vaginal infection by *Candida albicans, Trichomonas vaginalis,* or organisms causing bacterial vaginosis	(h) total cholesterol
(9) detects minute quantities of fecal blood	(i) VDRL or rapid plasma reagin

◆ CHAPTER 8 ◆

SEXUALITY CONCERNS

CHAPTER OVERVIEW

The sexual health of the childbearing family and its members is vital to their functioning throughout the life cycle. The nurse who works with such families must address sensitive sexuality concerns, possess a thorough understanding of sexuality and various sexual practices, and recognize any personal attitudes that could create barriers to good client rapport. To prepare the nurse to respond to a client's sexual health care needs, Chapter 8 summarizes the physiology of female and male sexual responses, explaining their clinical significance. It discusses how various psychological, social, and cultural factors affect sexuality and its changes throughout the life cycle. The chapter highlights the impact of the childbearing cycle on sexuality and specifies the sexual history-taking skills that help the nurse collect data for a comprehensive assessment. It reviews commonly encountered sexual dysfunctions and applies the steps of the nursing process to a client seeking sexual health care.

STUDENT ACTIVITIES

To test your familiarity with the information in this chapter, complete the following activities.

Clinical simulations

1. Five months into her first pregnancy, Barbara Woolston tells the nurse during a prenatal visit that she and her husband now are more active sexually than ever. She asks if this is normal. How should the nurse reply?

2. Beth and John Garrity arrive together for Beth's 6-week postpartal examination after the birth of their first child, Derrick. They tell the nurse-midwife that they have settled into a manageable routine with Derrick and gradually are adjusting to life with a neonate. Beth tells the nurse-midwife that her episiotomy healed completely about 1 month after her uncomplicated normal vaginal delivery; also, her lochia stopped around that time. However, despite her normal recover y, she confides that she is reluctant to resume intercourse. John complains that Beth "never seems to be in the mood" for sex. He also worries that because of the episiotomy scar, he might hurt her during intercourse. Describe how the nurse-midwife can use the nursing process to enhance this couple's sexual activity.

Multiple choice

3. An individual's sexual response is *not* influenced by:
(a) psychological state
(b) degree of myotonia

(c) illness or medication
(d) sexual motivation

4. In a parent effectiveness class attended by parents of preschoolers, the nurse educator discusses aspects of sexuality established in early childhood. Which of the following topics would *not* be discussed in this class?
(a) basic sexual identity
(b) stimuli for sexual arousal
(c) sexual fears and preoccupations
(d) the central conflict posed by sexual intimacy

Study questions

5. Briefly describe the effects of vasocongestion in response to sexual stimulation.

6. How did Masters and Johnson contribute to our early understanding of the common physiologic phases of the sexual response cycle? How does the more current approach toward the physiologic phases of the sexual response cycle for mulated by the American Psychiatric Association differ from the original work of Masters and Johnson?

7. Which aspects of sexuality should serve as the focus of a human growth and development course for junior high school students?

8. What suggestions can the nurse offer to elderly clients to help them maintain a positive sexual self-concept and an active sex life after the climacteric?

9. When taking a client's sexual history, the nurse should use open-ended questions that convey acceptance rather than judgment. Rephrase the three screening history questions suggested by Woods (see text page 158) so that they elicit insightful or thoughtful responses rather than a simple yes or no answer.

10. Given that the range of sexual normality is hard to define, which guidelines should the nurse use when evaluating a particular sexual behavior during client counseling?

11. List the four major categories of sexual dysfunctions.

12. The PLISSIT model is an appropriate intervention strategy for the nurse to use when providing sexual counseling for clients experiencing sexual problems. Briefly describe how the nurse can intervene at each of the four levels of this model.

13. Briefly discuss the roles that a nurse might serve when providing sexual health care.

Fill in the blank

14. Previously known as impotence, male sexual disorder is characterized by partial or complete failure to ____________, accompanied by lack of a subjective sense of pleasure during sex.

15. ___________ refers to recurrent or persistent genital pain before, during, or after sexual intercourse.

16. A woman with vaginismus experiences involuntary spasms of the musculature of the ___________, which interfere with intercourse.

17. Sexual desire refers to the frequency with which a person wishes to have sexual relations, whereas arousal is the ___________ of sexual excitement, as ascertained by the client's self-report.

Matching terms and definitions

18. Match each definition in the left column with the corresponding term in the right column.

(1) ongoing process of recognizing, accepting, and expressing oneself as a sexual being	(a) androgyny
(2) combination of male and female characteristics in the same individual	(b) libido
(3) period during the sexual response cycle when vasocongestion and myotonia peak	(c) orgasmic phase
(4) time after an orgasm when a man cannot experience restimulation and orgasm	(d) refractory period
(5) psychic energy or instinctual drive associated with sexual desire, pleasure, or creativity	(e) sexuality
(6) swelling, as when the penis or breasts swell during sexual activity	(f) tumescence

Values clarification

This exercise can help the nurse become a more effective sexual health advocate by increasing awareness of personal values, enhancing self-acceptance as a sexual being, and improving communication skills with clients. Complete each of the following sentences with the first thought that comes to mind.

19. When I think about discussing sexuality issues with a client, I feel...

20. Sexual behavior that clashes with my own code of ethics or morality makes me feel...

21. The areas of sexuality that cause me to feel guilty are...

22. When I was growing up, the messages I received about my body were...

23. When it came to sexual discussions or asking my family a question about sex, it was clear to me that ...

24. I first learned about sex when....

25. When I first learned about sex, I felt...

26. The most disturbing sexual experience I ever had was...

27. My religion tells me that sex is...

28. The thing I enjoy most about my sexuality is...

29. When I think about my sexuality in the future, I...

30. Discussing sexual health matters with adolescents makes me feel ...

What did you just discover about your attitudes, feelings, and beliefs about sexuality? How might these attitudes, feelings, and beliefs affect your comfort level and professional competence in addressing your clients' sexual health concerns?

◆ CHAPTER 9 ◆

FAMILY PLANNING

CHAPTER OVERVIEW

Because nurses have taken on increasingly complex, sophisticated responsibilities in providing family planning services, the nurse must be knowledgeable about all available family planning methods. Chapter 9 outlines the goals and principles of family planning, which provide a framework to guide nursing care. It describes the wide range of available contraceptive methods, offering strategies for teaching clients how to use these methods. It highlights the nursing process, demonstrating how the proper use of assessment data, nursing diagnosis, planning, implementation, and evaluation help ensure effective family planning care.

STUDENT ACTIVITIES

To test your familiarity with the information in this chapter, complete the following activities.

Clinical simulations

1. Marilynn, a single, 19-year-old college student, visits the campus health center to obtain birth control information. During the nursing assessment, she states that she is in good health and has no significant medical or surgical history. However, she mentions that her mother has high blood pressure, which she must take medication to control. Marilynn's last Pap smear, taken 1 year ago, was negative. She reports that she had an abortion 3 years ago and was treated for chlamydia, a sexually transmitted disease (STD), last year. List at least five other essential components of Marilynn's health history that the nurse must collect to help determine Marilynn's best choice of contraception.

2. Marilynn reveals that she has been sexually active for nearly 4 years. She states that although she has had multiple partners while at college, she has been dating one man steadily for 2 months. Of the following birth control methods, which one should the nurse discourage Marilynn from using? Explain your answer.
   (a) oral contraceptive
   (b) diaphragm
   (c) condoms with contraceptive foam
   (d) sympto-thermal method

3. Marilynn prefers an oral contraceptive as a birth control method. Which other birth control method should you advise her to use in conjunction with an oral contraceptive to protect her reproductive health? Explain your answer.

4. How should you go about teaching Marilynn about the low-dose estrogen contraceptive that the physician has prescribed?

5. Pat and Jim Brown, a childless couple in their mid-thirties, are planning a pregnancy within 1 year. Which of the following contraceptive methods is contraindicated for them? Explain your answer.
(a) oral contraceptive
(b) diaphragm
(c) contraceptive sponge
(d) intrauterine device

6. Colleen Green and Bill O'Rourke, devout Roman Catholics, are engaged. During a gynecologic visit, Colleen requests information on natural family planning, stating that she and Bill want to wait 1 year before conceiving their first child. Which five natural family planning methods should the nurse present as options for this couple?

7. Cherise is preparing for a vacuum curettage to terminate her pregnancy in its sixth week. When providing anticipatory guidance about her recovery, which topics should the nurse review with her?

8. Susan and Ernie are considering a tubal ligation now that their children are grown and they are certain they do not want another child. Describe the preoperative counseling the nurse should provide.

Multiple choice

9. Of the following principles, which one is *not* a sound guideline to follow when counseling a client seeking help with family planning?
(a) Every client has the right to receive the necessary information to make an informed decision.
(b) Information should be provided in an open, nonjudgmental, respectful manner free of the professional's personal bias.
(c) Family planning is a private, personal choice that affects only the couple involved.
(d) Identification and treatment of sexually transmitted diseases are important components of family planning.

10. Of the following descriptions, three apply to both the diaphragm and cervical cap. Which one applies only to the cervical cap?
(a) is a flexible rubber device used with spermicide
(b) acts as a mechanical barrier to sperm
(c) does not alter the body's metabolic or physiologic processes
(d) can be inserted 8 hours before intercourse and requires no spermicide reapplication before repeated intercourse.

Study questions

11. State one way in which a nurse can carry out each of the following roles effectively when working with a client seeking help with family planning: teacher, counselor, advocate, and researcher.

12. Identify the five major types of contraceptive methods.

13. Each contraceptive method has advantages and disadvantages. The left column below lists contraceptive methods; the right column lists advantages and disadvantages. Indicate which contraceptive method each advantage or disadvantage applies to by placing the

appropriate initial (or initials) after it. (Some advantages and disadvantages may apply to more than one method).

OC: oral contraceptives	(a) can be obtained over the counter in various colors, textures, and contours
CC: cervical cap	(b) necessitates physical dexterity and touching of genitals during insertion and withdrawal
D: diaphragm	(c) helps to regulate the menstrual cycle and decrease the menstrual flow, reducing the risk of anemia
C: condom	(d) does not alter the body's hormone balance
VS: vaginal spermicides	(e) decreases the risk of STDs
CS: contraceptive sponge	(f) usually cannot be detected by either partner during intercourse, if properly inserted
NFP: natural family planning	(g) has the lowest failure rate of any nonsurgical contraceptive method
IUD: intrauterine device	(h) increases the risk of monilia vaginitis
	(i) can cause an allergic reaction in either partner
	(j) may break or come apart during removal and may be hard to retrieve
	(k) restricts sexual spontaneity during the client's fertile period and requires extended periods of abstinence
	(l) may cause dysmenorrhea and increased menstrual flow after insertion

14. When providing complete information about contraceptive methods to a couple seeking family planning guidance, what aspects of each method must the nurse describe?

15. List at least three reasons why a client might wish to terminate her pregnancy.

16. Explain why the nurse who assists clients with family planning must be familiar with personal beliefs and attitudes about family planning.

Matching terms and definitions

17. Match each definition in the left column with the corresponding term in the right column.

(1) flexible, dome-shaped, rubber device with a thick rim that contains a spring; used with a spermicide	(a) abortion
(2) spontaneous or induced removal of products of conception before the second trimester of pregnancy	(b) basal body temperature method
(3) natural contraceptive method in which the male withdraws his penis from the vagina immediately before ejaculation	(c) cervical cap
(4) Japanese seaweed used in some abortions to dilate the cervix	(d) coitus interruptus
(5) abdominal incision above the pubis through which female sterilization can be performed	(e) condom
(6) painful menstruation; possible contraindication to IUD use	(f) contraceptive sponge
(7) natural contraceptive method that predicts a woman's fertile period by analyzing the length of previous menstrual cycles	(g) diaphragm
(8) plastic device that may contain copper or hormones; is placed inside the uterine cavity to prevent pregnancy	(h) dilatation and curettage
(9) natural contraceptive method that predicts a woman's fertile period by monitoring her daily morning body temperature	(i) dysmenorrhea
(10) chemical substance that kills sperm; available in contraceptive foams, jellies, and suppositories	(j) hysteroscopy
(11) male surgical sterilization method that involves ligating or cauterizing part of the vas deferens	(k) intrauterine device

(12) natural contraceptive method that predicts a woman's fertile period based on signs and symptoms of ovulation, including basal body temperature, cervical mucus changes, and mittelschmerz — (l) laminaria

(13) series of hormone tablets that inhibits ovulation — (m) minilaparotomy

(14) surgical method of pregnancy interruption that requires cervical dilatation and suction to evacuate the uterine contents — (n) oral contraceptive

(15) flexible, cup-shaped rubber device that fits over the cervix; used with a spermicide to act as a sperm barrier — (o) rhythm method

(16) surgical method of pregnancy termination that requires cervical dilatation and uterine scraping with a metal curette — (p) spermicide

(17) visual examination of the uterus through an illuminated tube that has been passed through the vagina; achieves sterilization by occluding the fallopian tubes with silicone — (q) sympto-thermal method

(18) thin sheath of rubber or some other material that is worn over the erect penis during intercourse to prevent sperm from entering the vagina — (r) vacuum curettage

(19) doughnut-shaped device containing spermicide and made from a soft, synthetic material — (s) vasectomy

◆ CHAPTER 10 ◆

FERTILITY AND INFERTILITY

CHAPTER OVERVIEW

Bearing and rearing children are developmental tasks that most people assume they will undertake as adults; many choose to plan the number and timing of their pregnancies. Clients ready to have a child may seek preconception counseling to ensure optimal conditions for conception and pregnancy; clients who have had trouble conceiving may seek help to overcome the problem or to cope with the anxiety or despondency they feel. Chapter 10 reviews the essentials of female and male fertility, preparing the nurse to work with couples who desire preconception planning, who wish to learn about conception, or who have had trouble conceiving. It surveys cultural myths and beliefs surrounding fertility and provides interventions to promote preconception health and minimize pregnancy risk factors for prepregnancy planning in fertile couples. Next, the chapter presents the etiology of female and male infertility, describes diagnostic tests that determine the cause of infertility, and explores medical treatments for infertility. It emphasizes nursing responsibilities for clients who have concerns about their fertility or infertility.

STUDENT ACTIVITIES

To test your familiarity with the information in this chapter, complete the following activities.

Clinical simulations

1. Linda, age 39, is a single nulliparous client who visits the clinic "for a general physical to make sure everything is all right, so I can get pregnant again." During the health history interview, she states that she works at a dry-cleaning plant, where she cleans and processes clothing. Her income is marginal, and she is not eligible for the company's health insurance plan. She had two early elective abortions, 10 and 12 years earlier, without complications; less than 1 year ago, she miscarried. Linda is 25% over her ideal weight, takes medication to control hypertension, and smokes one and a half packs of cigarettes a day. Her only sibling is a younger brother; she describes him as "a slow learner who will never be able to live on his own. He may be mentally retarded." Her father also has hypertension; her mother has diabetes and must take oral hypoglycemics. Based on Linda's history, identify at least five risk factors that place her at high risk for conception and pregnancy complications.

2. Which other historical data should the nurse collect to complete Linda's preconception health assessment?

3. Linda says she wants to become pregnant now because "my time is running out and my mother wants grandchildren." Her steady boy-

friend, Andy, has two children from a previous marriage. The nurse formulates a nursing diagnosis of *family coping: potential for growth, related to impending pregnancy*. Which counseling strategies should the nurse use to help Linda achieve optimal preconception health?

4. Roxanna and Alfredo Bonares, married for 2 years, have decided that they are ready to start a family. Roxanna, age 28, is a bookkeeper with no previous pregnancies; Alfredo, age 29, is a financial analyst. Which five major topics should the nurse include in health promotion strategies when guiding this couple toward optimal preconception health?

5. Melissa, age 27, and Stuart, age 34, have been married for 9 years. Both are devoted to their careers. After trying unsuccessfully to conceive for 3 years, they have decided to seek medical help at the urging of Melissa's mother. The nurse at the infertility clinic notices that although Melissa and Stuart are bright and attractive, they seem depressed and self-effacing when discussing their disappointment over not having children. For this reason, the nurse suspects that they have disturbances in self-concept and body image. Describe possible feelings associated with such disturbances in an infertile couple.

6. The nurse has collected a thorough history on Melissa and Stuart, and an infertility specialist has conducted their physical examinations and ordered appropriate diagnostic tests. What role will the nurse subsequently play in their care?

7. Karen, a 39-year-old investment broker, and her husband Clive, a 35-year-old attorney, have gone through an extensive infertility workup. The findings reveal that although Karen ovulates regularly and Clive produces adequate sperm, Karen's cervical mucus creates a hostile environment for sperm survival. Consequently, the physician recommends the gamete intrafallopian transfer (GIFT) procedure. After making a nursing diagnosis of ***knowledge deficit related to infertility treatments***, the nurse should provide what anticipatory guidance to Karen and Clive to help them better understand this procedure?

8. Karen and Clive have stated that one of their goals is to cope with the stress of the GIFT procedure successfully. Based on this goal, how should the nurse state evaluation findings for nursing care provided for Karen and Clive?

Study questions

9. State three possible reasons for the increasing incidence of infertility in the United States.

10. Over the centuries, cultural myths and beliefs regarding fertility have developed. Even today, such myths and beliefs may exert a subtle influence on a client's self-esteem and perceptions about her capacity for childbearing. Give at least two examples of cultural symbols of fertility or cultural rituals used to promote fertility.

11. Provide a brief definition of infertility.

12. Identify three possible causes for each of the following factors associated with female, male, and combined infertility.
Factors associated with female infertility:
- structural changes in the uterus
- anovulation secondary to ovarian failure or faulty hormonal stimulation

Factors associated with male infertility:
- spermatogenesis
- reproductive tract structures

Factors associated with combined infertility:
- alteration in sexual function

13. What are some common effects of infertility evaluation and treatment on a couple's sexuality? What are some related feelings reported by couples who have undergone such evaluation and treatment?

Fill in the blank

14. In __________, oocytes are removed from the woman's body, mixed with her partner's sperm, incubated, then placed in the uterus.

15. The drug __________ induces ovulation by triggering increased production of follicle-stimulating hormone (FSH).

16. In the __________ procedure, oocytes and sperm are transferred into the distal end of the fallopian tube to allow in vivo fertilization.

17. Simulated instillation of sperm into the vagina for conception is called __________.

18. __________ and __________ are two substances that reduce oligopspermia chemically by increasing follicle-stimulating hormone.

True or false

19. Only about half of infertile couples can be treated successfully.
❑ True ❑ False

20. In at least 40% of infertile couples, the exact cause of infertility cannot be determined.
❑ True ❑ False

21. In most cases, infertility stems from male hormonal or structural factors.
❑ True ❑ False

22. Nonreproductive factors, such as occupational hazards or drug use, may cause infertility in males or females.
❑ True ❑ False

Matching terms and definitions

23. Match each definition in the left column with the corresponding term in the right column.

(1) anterior pituitary hormone that stimulates follicular growth in women and promotes spermatogenesis in men	(a) basal body temperature
(2) stretchiness of the cervical mucus at ovulation	(b) endometrial biopsy
(3) expulsion of an ovum from the ovary upon spontaneous rupture of a mature follicle	(c) follicle-stimulating hormone
(4) X-ray film of the uterus and fallopian tubes to detect uterine abnormalities and assess tubal patency	(d) hysterosalpingography
(5) abnormally low number of sperm in the semen	(e) laparoscopy
(6) visual examination of the internal abdomen through an illuminated tube inserted through an abdominal incision, performed to assess a woman's reproductive organs for causes of infertility	(f) oligospermia
(7) test in which a sample taken from the uterine lining is analyzed to determine the condition of the endometrium and to help identify the phase of the menstrual cycle	(g) ovulation
(8) lowest body temperature of a healthy individual while awake; can be assessed for daily changes that predict a woman's fertile period	(h) spinnbarkeit
(9) assessment of sperm survival in the cervical mucus after sexual intercourse	(i) endometriosis
(10) abnormal gynecologic condition in which endometrial tissue grows and functions outside the uterine cavity	(j) postcoital examination

◆ CHAPTER 11 ◆

GENETICS AND GENETIC DISORDERS

CHAPTER OVERVIEW

Once a woman who desires pregnancy conceives, she and her family begin to anticipate the birth of a healthy neonate possessing full intellectual and physical potential. Unfortunately, not all neonates escape birth defects or genetic diseases. Ideally, the nurse caring for the childbearing or child-rearing family assesses genetic risk factors during preconception counseling and teaches prospective parents about the potential for genetic disorders. The nurse also provides information, makes referrals for evaluation and possible treatment of a potential genetic disorder, and promotes a healthy prenatal environment to maximize pregnancy outcome. After the birth of a neonate with an unexpected genetic or congenital disorder, the nurse provides support and information to the family. These nursing responsibilities necessitate a basic understanding of genetics and genetic disorders. Chapter 11 provides this knowledge base. It explains the transference of genetic information during conception and embryonic and fetal development—a crucial step in growth and development. After describing such concepts as genes, chromosomes, deoxyribonucleic acid (DNA), and cell division by mitosis and meiosis, it summarizes major causes of genetic disorders—including monogenic factors, chromosomal abnormalities, and multifactorial influences. The chapter also reviews the diagnostic tests used to detect risk factors and genetic or congenital disorders.

STUDENT ACTIVITIES

To test your familiarity with the information in this chapter, complete the following activities.

Clinical simulations

1. In her late twenties, Ginger Neeson is diagnosed with Huntington's chorea, a degenerative neuromuscular disease that claimed the life of her father just before she began to show signs. Which type of inheritance pattern does this monogenic (single-gene) hereditary disorder exhibit? Based on the inheritance pattern, what are the chances that Ginger's two siblings also have inherited Huntington's chorea?

2. Sherrelle and Justin Simpson, a Black couple, arrive at the prenatal clinic for their initial pregnancy evaluation. During the health history interview, Justin reveals that he has sickle cell trait. The nurse practitioner then orders a sickle cell screening test for Sherrelle, a primigravid client age 19 who has never been tested. Explain why the nurse practitioner orders this test.

3. Bill Johnson is color blind; prenatal screening shows that his wife, Gerri, is not a carrier of this disorder. After the birth of their son, the nurse assures the Johnsons that their son will not be color blind. What is the basis for the nurse's statement?

4. Terry McCabe, age 4, has a mild form of neurofibromatosis, an autosomal dominant disorder. His two older siblings do not have the disease. His maternal grandfather had a more serious form of neurofibromatosis, although he never was diagnosed appropriately. When Terry's parents, Jennie and Ralph, visit the genetic clinic for preconception counseling for their fourth child, they ask the nurse why Jennie and her two other children do not have this disorder. What are some factors the nurse might mention when explaining why neurofibromatosis and other autosomal disorders sometimes are difficult to trace?

Study questions

5. Briefly describe the mechanism for somatic cell division that is responsible for growth, development, and maintenance throughout life.

6. Describe the process of meiosis (gametogenesis) in the male.

7. Explain how fertilization occurs on a cellular level.

8. Male and female sex chromosomes within each reproductive cell commonly are indicated by letters. Provide the proper letters for the male and female primary diploid cells (spermatocyte and oocyte).

9. What are the three major factors that result in genetic disorders?

10. Name the inheritance pattern that occurs in monogenic disorders in which an abnormal gene exists on the X chromosome and this abnormal gene is transmitted by only one parent.

11. What is a three-generation pedigree? How is it used in genetic counseling? Which information should it include?

12. When referring a couple for genetic counseling based in their preconception history, what should the nurse tell them to expect from this type of counseling?

13. Although genetic counseling requires special preparation, the nurse can participate as a member of the clinical team. Identify at least five of the many roles the nurse can fulfill when working with a family requiring genetic counseling.

Fill in the blank

14. The ____________ is the biological unit of heredity, containing information that determines the unique biological and behavioral characteristics of each human being.

15. ____________ are microscopic, threadlike chemical structures within the cell nuclei containing genetic information in a linear sequence.

16. Varying combinations of nitrogen bases on each strand of ____________ produce genetic differences among people.

17. In somatic cells, division occurs through the process of ____________; in reproductive cells, division occurs by ____________.

18. Meiosis produces specialized reproductive cells called ____________.

19. An observable expression of genetically determined traits (such as blue eyes or red hair) is called a phenotype, whereas the total genetic constitution is referred to as a ____________.

True or false

20. Chromosomal abnormalities may be involved in approximately half of all spontaneous abortions.
❑ True ❑ False

21. Major congenital abnormalities affect 2% to 3% of all neonates.
❑ True ❑ False

22. Abnormal chromosomal rearrangements tend to manifest consistently, causing easily identifiable signs at birth.
❑ True ❑ False

23. Because autosomes outnumber sex chromosomes by 44 to 2, most monogenic disorders involve autosomes.
❑ True ❑ False

24. Chromosomal abnormalities specifically refer only to those related to distorted numerical patterns.
❑ True ❑ False

25. Mutations are permanent, inheritable changes in gene sequence that occur rarely.
❑ True ❑ False

Matching terms and definitions

26. Hundreds of genetic disorders can be diagnosed prenatally. Some prenatal tests are used for screening; others are diagnostic. Nurses working in all areas of maternal and neonatal care must be familiar with these tests in case a client requires such testing or needs a referral for it. Match each genetic test shown in the left column with the corresponding description in the right column.

(1) radiography	(a) photographing and arranging of fetal chromosomes by number to check for numerical and structural abnormalities; used when a fetal chromosomal abnormality is suspected
(2) chorionic villus sampling	(b) maternal blood test that measures a glycoprotein normally excreted by the fetus into the amniotic fluid and absorbed through the placenta into the maternal bloodstream; used to screen for fetal neural tube defects
(3) fetoscopy	(c) biopsy sample of placental tissue removed transcervically 9 to 12 weeks after the last menstrual period; identifies all common chromosomal disorders in the fetus except neural tube defects
(4) ultrasonography	(d) X-ray visualization of fetal skeletal or limb malformations
(5) karyotyping	(e) fetal imaging test involving sound waves; used to detect gross fetal structural abnormalities or guide certain prenatal diagnostic procedures
(6) amniocentesis	(f) fetal visualization via a fiberoptic scope inserted through the abdominal wall
(7) maternal serum alpha fetoprotein test	(g) amniotic fluid withdrawal via needle aspiration; allows chromosomal analysis and measurement of amniotic fluid alpha fetoprotein and acetylcholinesterase levels

◆ CHAPTER 12 ◆

INFECTIOUS DISORDERS

CHAPTER OVERVIEW

Infectious disorders that affect a woman's sexual health, reproductive health, or genitourinary system are relatively common in the United States. Certain infections with serious long-term consequences are increasing in incidence; some can cause infertility or even lead to death. Infectious disorders also may take an emotional toll, causing social stigma that affects a woman's sexuality. Chapter 12 discusses the most common infectious disorders that influence women's genitourinary, gynecologic, and reproductive health. It discusses the causes, clinical findings, and treatments for each infection, providing the knowledge base the nurse needs to help the client understand the disease and to provide emotional as well as physical support.

STUDENT ACTIVITIES

To test your familiarity with the information in this chapter, complete the following activities.

Clinical simulations

1. Anne, a 19-year-old college student, comes to the health center complaining of a thick, white, curdy, odorless vaginal discharge accompaniedby vaginal itching and burning. During the nursing history interview, she reveals that she recently took an antibiotic after oral surgery and currently is under stress from her final examinations. She has been eating more sweets than usual because of anxiety; her appetite otherwise has been minimal. The nurse practitioner diagnoses candidiasis, a form of vaginitis. Explain why.

2. Gina, age 25, calls her gynecologist's office to request that the gynecologist prescribe "something for my yeast infection" and call in the prescription by telephone to her pharmacy. The nurse who speaks with Gina questions her further, eliciting a history of a thin, yellowish-gray vaginal discharge with a "fishy" odor. Based on this history, the nurse suggests that Gina come in for evaluation so that the gynecologist can identify the causative organism. Of the following infections, which one should the nurse suspect as the cause of Gina's symptoms?
   (a) candidiasis
   (b) trichomoniasis
   (c) bacterial vaginosis
   (d) pelvic inflammatory disease (PID)

3. Brenda, age 18, comes to the family planning clinic because she f ound out that her boyfriend is "sleeping around" and thinks she might have caught an infection from him. She describes a thick, yel-

low vaginal discharge and painful urination that began a few days earlier. She states that she had chills and fever the previous evening and reports increasing lower abdominal cramps. Physical examination reveals a temperature of 100.4° F (38° C); a pulse of 92 beats/minute; blood pressure of 100/60 mm Hg; and a respiratory rate of 24 breaths/minute. Brenda's abdomen is tender to palpation in the suprapubic area. Speculum examination shows a purulent cervical and vaginal discharge; bimanual palpation reveals cervical motion and uterine tenderness. Based on these findings, the physician tentatively diagnoses PID. Which laboratory studies should the nurse expect the physician to order? Describe the purpose of each test.

4. Donna, a single client age 22, comes to the emergency department complaining of a sudden high fever (103° F). She has influenza-like signs and symptoms and reports that she feels "very sick." During the nursing history interview, she points to an unusual red, spotty rash on her palms, which she said began the previous day, and describes increasing muscle pain and weakness. Her menstrual history is normal; she is on day 3 of her regular 5-day, moderate-flow menstrual cycle. She is sexually active with her steady boyfriend and uses a contraceptive sponge for birth control. Based on Donna's signs and symptoms, which of the following infections should the nurse suspect?
   (a) secondary syphilis
   (b) toxic shock syndrome (TSS)
   (c) pelvic inflammatory disease
   (d) pyelonephritis

5. Cyndy, a 26-year-old newlywed, comes to the health clinic complaining of severe pain and burning on urination for the past 2 days. Her symptoms caused such severe discomfort that she and her husband had to cut their honeymoon short. She states that she developed lower back discomfort this morning and saw blood in her urine before coming to the clinic. Her gynecologic, menstrual, and past medical histories are unremarkable. She and her husband delayed intercourse until after marriage; she uses a diaphragm for contraception.

   Based on further history findings, physical examination, and laboratory studies, the physician diagnoses cystitis. List six suggestions the nurse could make to help Cyndy prevent a recurrence of this common urinary tract infection.

6. During her initial prenatal visit, Myra, age 28, discloses her concern that she might have human immunodeficiency virus (HIV) infection. Which questions should the nurse ask to determine Myra's potential risk for this infection?

Study questions

7. What is the main difference between cystitis and pyelonephritis?

8. Of the medications commonly used to treat sexually transmitted diseases (STDs), which ones are contraindicated during pregnancy and breast-feeding?

9. Explain how the body maintains a normal vaginal environment to help prevent bacterial infection.

10. Which organisms typically cause PID? What are the potential effects of PID on reproductive health?

11. List six general goals for the nurse providing care for a client with an infectious disorder.

12. Name four predisposing factors for TSS.

13. What is the rationale for consistent use of universal precautions for infection control?

14. What essential areas should the nurse explore when obtaining a complete health history for a client who may have an infectious disorder?

15. In a client who is at high risk for HIV infection, the nurse should stay alert for which signs and symptoms?

16. The nurse should include which topics when teaching a client how to prevent a recurrence of candidiasis?

17. Describe some important information the nurse should cover when counseling a client with a negative enzyme-linked immunosorbent assay (ELISA) test result.

Fill in the blank

18. ____________ manifests as a thin, bubbly, yellow-green, malodorous vaginal discharge accompanied by moderate to severe vulvar pruritus.

19. Painful genital blisters that develop into shallow ulcers after a prodrome of influenza-like signs and symptoms indicate ____________ infection.

20. In ____________, one or more painless chancres appear on the genitals, anus, or lips; these chancres break down into indurated ulcers that disappear in about ____________ weeks.

21. Soft, fleshy, painless, wartlike growths in the anogenital area signal ____________ or ____________.

22. In ____________, papular lesions arise in sites where mites burrow, and extreme pruritus occurs along body creases.

3. ____________ is characterized by tiny white specks near the base of hair shafts that resist removal.

True or false

24. Chlamydia is the most common STD in the United States.
❑ True ❑ False

25. Herpes genitalis can be transmitted only through sexual intercourse.
❑ True ❑ False

26. Although HIV has been isolated in various body fluids, it is transmitted only through blood, semen, vaginal secretions, and possibly breast milk.
❑ True ❑ False

27. Anal intercourse is especially likely to cause HIV transmission.
❑ True ❑ False

28. Most people with HIV infection can be identified by their appearance.
❑ True ❑ False

29. A pregnant woman with HIV infection may pass the infection to her fetus in utero or to her neonate via breast milk.
❑ True ❑ False

Matching related elements

30. Nurses must be familiar with the medications commonly prescribed to treat STDs. Match the STD in the left column with each medication that is routinely prescribed for it, shown in the right column. (A medication may be prescribed for more than one STD.)

(1) chlamydia	(a) ceftriaxone sodium plus doxycycline
(2) trichomoniasis	(b) acyclovir sodium
(3) herpes genitalis	(c) podophyllum resin or trichloroacetic acid
(4) pediculosis pubis	(d) metronidazole
(5) gonorrhea	(e) doxycycline hyclate or tetracycline
(6) syphilis	(f) lindane shampoo
(7) condylomata acuminata	(g) penicillin G benzathine
(8) scabies	

◆ CHAPTER 13 ◆

GYNECOLOGIC DISORDERS

CHAPTER OVERVIEW

Disorders of the female reproductive system can have profound physical, emotional, and sexual implications, affecting a client's health, self-image, and intimate relationships. Some disorders represent normal female variations; others reflect the effects of aging, infection, or serious disease. To provide effective care for a client with a gynecologic disorder, the nurse must have the advanced knowledge and clinical skills to recognize the disorder early, make appropriate referrals for prompt treatment, and remain sensitive to the psychosocial issues involved. Chapter 13 describes the most commonly encountered gynecologic disorders—breast disorders, menstrual disorders, pelvic support disorders, and gynecologic cancer. After defining each disorder, it shows how to apply the nursing process when providing client care. The chapter highlights emotional support measures and client teaching.

STUDENT ACTIVITIES

To test your familiarity with the information in this chapter, complete the following activities.

Clinical simulations

1. Mildred Kayro, age 53, is a divorced nulliparous client who comes to the health center after discovering a painless lump in her breast. As the nurse takes her health history, Mrs. Kayro reveals that both her mother and maternal grandmother had breast cancer. Her general health is good; however, she was unable to conceive because of anovulatory menstrual cycles related to obesity. She states that she knows she should lose weight but loves to eat and is especially fond of steaks and ice cream. Identify some factors in Mrs. Kayro's history that increase her risk for breast cancer.

2. As the nurse obtains her health history during her annual gynecologic examination, Claudine Shelby, age 49, tearfully reveals that she discovered a lump nearly a year ago when examining her breasts. The nurse asks why she did not seek medical evaluation right away. What are some possible reasons for Mrs. Shelby's delay?

3. During her annual gynecologic examination, Dianne, a 39-year-old multiparous client, asks the nurse how she can cope better with the mood swings she experiences every month just before her period starts. She reports that she feels bloated and has insomnia during this time; lately, the problem has worsened and has begun to upset her husband and their two teenage daughters. How should the

nurse explain this cyclic pattern to Dianne? What measures should the nurse suggest to alleviate her symptoms?

4. Melissa Charles, age 26, is a single, sexually active client who visits the nurse practitioner for her yearly gynecologic examination. The physical examination reveals nodular and diffusely grainy breast tissue bilaterally, accompanied by slight tenderness to the touch. Noting that Ms. Charles is in the last half of her menstrual cycle, the nurse practitioner suspects fibrocystic breast changes. Briefly describe some common treatments the nurse practitioner might recommend.

5. Alicia, a high school sophomore, visits the school nurse complaining of severe menstrual cramps. When teaching Alicia about measures that may help relieve her dysmenorrhea, the nurse should cover what topics?

6. Fiona Clark, a 23-year-old nulligravid client, tells Marybeth Andrews, the nurse practitioner at the health center, that she found a small "knot" in her left breast during a breast self-examination (BSE). On assessment, Marybeth determines that the mass is approximately 1 cm, round, rubbery yet firm, discrete, relatively mobile, and nontender. Fiona has no family history of breast cancer. Marybeth should suspect which condition? Explain your answer.

7. Several days after her diagnosis of uterine cancer, Lara Derrickson asks the nurse to discuss the various treatment options she is considering. Explain how Mrs. Derrickson can benefit from such a discussion, and describe the nurse's role in providing information about her disease and its treatment.

8. Sharon Thomas, age 47, has just returned to her hospital room after a modified radical mastectomy. Provide at least five short-term and two long-term nursing goals for her postoperative care.

Multiple choice

9. Primary amenorrhea is associated with which of the following?
   (a) nutritional factors (such as anorexia)
   (b) oral contraceptives
   (c) congenital defects
   (d) stress or anxiety

10. When teaching a client about colposcopy, the nurse should *not* include which of the following information? Explain your answer.
   (a) The procedure does not cause discomfort.
   (b) The procedure is performed between menstrual periods.
   (c) The procedure takes place in a physician's office or a clinic.
   (d) Acetic acid is used to wash the cervix for better visualization.

11. The second leading cause of death in women is:
   (a) uterine cancer
   (b) ovarian cancer
   (c) breast cancer
   (d) cervical cancer

12. The most common benign breast condition is:
    (a) fibroadenoma
    (b) fibrocystic breast changes
    (c) intraductal papilloma
    (d) duct ectasia

13. Which of the following factors does *not* increase a client's risk of cervical cancer?
    (a) multiple sex partners
    (b) smoking
    (c) use of a barrier contraceptive
    (d) sexual intercourse before age 18

Study questions

14. Explain why the nurse should encourage every client to perform a monthly BSE.

15. Identify some factors that may affect a client's perception of a particular gynecologic disorder.

16. What are the four standard medical treatments for breast cancer?

17. List at least five factors that influence the choice of treatment for breast cancer.

18. Identify the major warning signs of gynecologic cancer.

Matching terms and definitions

19. Match each definition in the left column with the corresponding glossary term in the right column.

(1) malignant tumor within surface epithelium that has not penetrated deeper tissues	(a) amenorrhea
(2) removal of one or both ovaries	(b) carcinoma in situ
(3) absence of menses	(c) cryosurgery
(4) treatment that destroys tissue by applying extreme cold	(d) cystocele
(5) X-ray used to detect tumors and other breast abnormalities	(e) dyspareunia
(6) uterine bleeding between menstrual periods	(f) endometriosis
(7) incision through the abdominal wall	(g) laparotomy
(8) descent of the uterus from its normal position in the pelvis	(h) mammography
(9) abdominal pain related to ovulation	(i) metrorrhagia

(10) painful or difficult intercourse	(j) mittleschmerz
(11) bladder protrusion through a weakness in the vaginal wall	(k) oophorectomy
(12) growth of endometrial tissue outside the uterine cavity	(l) uterine prolapse

◆ CHAPTER 14 ◆

VIOLENCE AGAINST WOMEN

CHAPTER OVERVIEW

Violence against women is a local, national, personal, and professional concern for nurses. Such violence takes many forms and may lead to serious, long-term psychological trauma. The nurse must provide all-encompassing care for the client who has survived violence, assessing and intervening appropriately for both physical and psychological trauma incurred. Besides providing a safe environment to protect the client and her rights, the nurse must establish a trusting relationship with her and assist with physical examinations. In some cases, the nurse also must ensure proper collection of laboratory data to test for sexually transmitted diseases (STDs) and provide evidence for criminal prosecution. Chapter 14 investigates the various types of violence committed against women, discusses the impact of violence, and describes the comprehensive nursing care required.

STUDENT ACTIVITIES

To test your familiarity with the information in this chapter, complete the following activities.

Clinical simulations

1. Wendy, age 26, is admitted to the emergency department with multiple contusions of the face and arms. During the nursing health history, she rarely makes eye contact and shows little emotion. She says her injuries occurred when she fell on the stairs while carrying groceries into the house. Wendy's neighbor brought her to the health care facility. Her husband, who arrives shortly after she does, hovers over her and seems annoyed that she requires medical care. Wendy appears passive and refuses to disclose more information about the incident. Which elements of Wendy's history suggest that she is the victim of abuse rather than the accident she described?

2. When Wendy returns to the clinic for follow-up care several days later, she seems more willing to talk. During the nursing assessment, she admits that her injuries occurred when her husband assaulted her after losing his temper. However, she quickly comes to his defense. "He didn't mean to hurt me," she explains. "He never does. Every once in a while, I do stupid things that make him angry, and then he explodes. He's so sorry he hurt me that he broke down and cried when we got home. He promised he wouldn't do it again. He really loves me." Provide a brief explanation for Wendy's rationalization of her husband's abuse.

3. Which phase of Walker's cycle of violence are Wendy and her husband apparently experiencing at this time? Briefly describe what happens during this phase.

4. During the past 6 months, Juanita, a 32-year-old mother of five, has visited the health clinic many times with vague somatic complaints. Seemingly stress-related, the complaints have never required special treatment. Juanita sometimes expresses concern for her husband, who "works so hard and never earns enough." Usually, she brings several of her children along for various health concerns. Today, however, she comes alone. Visibly shaken, she limps and has an extensive bruise on her right forearm, which she clutches to her side. The nurse determines that she may be the victim of physical abuse. Briefly summarize how to proceed with her during this visit.

5. As the physician examines Juanita, the nurse notices that she appears unusually disheveled and hesitates before answering questions. She moves slowly and indicates extreme pain when her right arm is examined. While helping Juanita remove her dress, the nurse sees large bruises on her right hip and shoulder and notes that she has extremely limited mobility and marked guarding. X-rays reveal a dislocated right shoulder and a spiral fracture of the radius.

   Because Juanita is uncomfortable and overwhelmed, she cannot set goals for her care at this time. She states only that her "accident" happened because her husband had been drinking and started an argument. After obtaining all the necessary data, the nurse formulates a nursing diagnosis of ***post-trauma response related to abuse***. Which nursing interventions might prove useful in helping Juanita obtain the assistance she needs?

6. Five weeks after this incident, Juanita visits the clinic again, showing further signs of abuse. The nurse becomes angry with her for staying with her husband, fearing that she will suffer further violence. How should the nurse proceed?

7. Gina, age 19, comes to the emergency department with bleeding from perineal trauma sustained while on a date with a man she met at college. Tearfully, she explains that "he wouldn't take no for an answer" after they returned to her apartment from a movie and had several glasses of wine. She states that he forced himself on her and that penile penetration occurred.

   After her discharge, Gina seems outwardly calm and subdued. She takes time off from school to put the event behind her, visiting a friend who does not know she has been raped. She resolves never to think about the rape again. Because she fears she will encounter the rapist at school, she transfers to another college closer to home, moving into a new apartment with a female roommate. Soon, however, she begins to feel increasingly anxious and cannot concentrate on her school work. She panics if her roommate comes home late or stays overnight at her boyfriend's apartment; over the next few months, she gains 40 pounds.

   Eventually, Gina visits the student health center complaining of increasingly irregular menses and difficulty sleeping. During the nursing history interview, she tells the nurse about the rape that occurred 6 months earlier and reports repeated violent nightmares about the attack. After obtaining this history, what condition should the nurse suspect as the cause of Gina's menstrual problems and insomnia? Briefly describe how this condition progresses.

8. June Carr, age 25, is brought to the emergency department after being raped outside her suburban home as she returned from work. Her husband is out of town on business; she was found by her neighbors, who heard her screaming and came to her aid as the assailant fled.

Some of the following statements reflect appropriate guidelines for a nurse providing legal advocacy for June; the remaining statements are inappropriate. Identify whether each statement is appropriate or inappropriate by placing an *A* or an *I* in the blank that precedes it. For each inappropriate guideline, explain your answer.
(a) Remain calm, professional, and detached so that June can take responsibility for notifying the police independently after she has been discharged from the health care facility.
(b) Ensure that the examining physician obtains informed consent before beginning treatment, and act as witness to June's consent.
(c) Stay with June during subsequent interviews to provide support and ensure that legal, law enforcement, and other individuals treat her properly.
(d) Be an active listener, and interject questions for police officers when appropriate, based on what you know about June's case.
(e) Ensure that no evidence is overlooked.
(f) Document the most relevant information on the appropriate hospital forms.
(g) Answer questions posed by June's neighbors, who anxiously await word on her condition.
(h) Provide June with general information about the legal process, and refer her for legal assistance.
(i) Arrange for a properly trained volunteer to accompany June to all police interviews and legal proceedings.

Study questions

9. Why should the nurse ask a rape survivor to describe the rape *before* collecting other health history data?

10. Explain the difference between sexual assault and rape.

11. Most facilities require the nurse caring for the rape survivor to document certain key informational categories—including pertinent medical and gynecologic history findings, result of mental status examination, physical assessment findings, and names of other people who questioned the client or were involved in her care. List three other categories that the nurse should document.

True or false

12. Rape carries a high risk of pregnancy.
❑ True ❑ False

13. Androgynous sex roles promote the abuse of women.
❑ True ❑ False

14. The risk of contracting an STD from rape is higher than the risk of pregnancy from rape.
❑ True ❑ False

15. Before assessing a rape survivor, the nurse should allow her to get comfortable and collect herself by going to the lavatory and freshening up, if she requests.
❑ True ❑ False

16. In most states, the laws provide no legal recourse for spousal rape.
❑ True ❑ False

Values clarification

Health care professionals who care for survivors of violence must be aware of their personal attitudes, feelings, and beliefs about such violence to ensure effective care. To help assess your attitudes, feelings, and beliefs, complete each of the following sentences with the first thought that comes to mind.

17. If someone I loved was abused by her spouse, I would react by ...

18. When I hear that a frustrated husband lost his temper because his wife spurned his sexual advances, I feel ...

19. I believe that a woman who stays with an abusive partner is ...

20. If I had to provide ongoing nursing care for a woman whose partner abused her repeatedly, I would feel ...

21. When I think about providing nursing care to an abused woman with her partner present, I ...

22. The notion of sexual violence makes me feel ...

23. When I hear someone say that a woman cannot be raped unless she is willing, I ...

24. When I imagine how I would respond if I were raped, I ...

25. When I hear someone say that women really mean "yes" when they say "no" to sex, I feel ...

What did you just discover about your attitudes, feelings, and beliefs about violence? How might these attitudes, feelings, and beliefs affect your comfort level and professional competence when providing care for survivors of violence?

◆ CHAPTER 15 ◆

WOMEN'S HEALTH-COMPROMISING BEHAVIORS

CHAPTER OVERVIEW

Dramatic shifts in women's roles and responsibilities over the past several decades have led to changes in their health behaviors, life-styles, and health needs. Chapter 15 explores the behaviors that compromise women's health—including nutritional concerns and substance abuse—and investigates the types of stress generated by the demanding lives that many women now lead. It explains how the nurse can assess and intervene for health-compromising behaviors and describes nursing interventions to help the client develop positive coping skills and health-promotion behaviors to reduce stress and prevent illness.

STUDENT ACTIVITIES

To test your familiarity with the information in this chapter, complete the following activities.

Clinical simulations

1. Sandra Garcia, age 23, comes to the health clinic for a routine gynecologic examination. She is 5′2″ tall and weighs 185 pounds. When counseling Sandra about her daily nutritional intake, the nurse should keep which socioeconomic and cultural factors in mind as potential influences on Sandra's food choices and eating patterns?

2. Sandra begins to cry when the nurse asks her how she feels about her weight. What is the likely underlying cause of her emotional upset over her obesity?

3. Sandra reports that she has been overweight since age 10. Given this historical data, should the nurse suspect that she has hyperplastic obesity or hypertrophic obesity? Does Sandra's obesity type make successful dieting easier or harder? Explain your answers.

4. Sandra explains that she has tried many crash diets but cannot stick with a diet once she loses the initial weight. Therefore, she gains all the lost weight back, plus additional weight. How should the nurse explain this cycle of weight loss and gain to Sandra?

5. Of the following treatments, the nurse might recommend which one for Sandra, who seems motivated to lose weight permanently? Explain your answer.
   - a medically supervised liquid diet
   - a nutritionally balanced, limited-calorie diet
   - intestinal bypass surgery
   - a non-calorie-counting diet that is high in protein and low in carbohydrates

6. Lila, age 32, is a single mother with three school-aged children. To support her family, she holds two jobs. She started smoking cigarettes in her junior year of high school; for the past few years, she has smoked a pack and a half daily. However, she recently decided to quit after reading about the long-term effects of smoking. During her visit to the physician for a routine gynecologic examination, Lila asks the nurse for advice on how to quit, expressing surprise over how difficult it is. What signs and symptoms of nicotine withdrawal should the nurse tell her to expect?

7. Mrs. Small comes to the health center to seek advice about her daughter Chris, age 16, who complains about being fat. The oldest of Mrs. Small's four children, Chris is a junior in high school and an academic overachiever. She is 5′6″ tall and weighs 92 pounds. Mrs. Small tells the nurse that during her freshman and sophomore years, Chris was 10 pounds overweight. When one of the most popular boys in her class asked her to the prom, she went on a crash diet, losing 20 pounds. She continues to follow a strict diet and has become obsessed with her daily exercise routine. She never seems satisfied with herself or her accomplishments. Mrs. Small say she is worried about how thin Chris has become and has begun to notice how little she eats. This has led to family fights during dinner. She states that her youngest child begs Chris to eat more; Chris always responds that she must be careful not to regain the weight she has lost. Identify the disorder affecting Chris, describe its possible causes, and list some methods the nurse could recommend to Mrs. Small for dealing with her daughter's problem.

8. Betty, age 34, comes to the health clinic for her first prenatal visit at 22 weeks' gestation. Her obstetric history reveals that she has delivered one full-term neonate and one preterm neonate who died; she also has had two abortions. During the nursing history interview, she reports that she smokes at least one pack of cigarettes a day. She also admits that she has smoked crack cocaine with her boyfriend, but says she stopped a few months ago when she discovered she was pregnant. What should the nurse tell Betty about the possible effects of smoking and cocaine use on her fetus?

Study questions

9. How have technological advances and changes within the food industry contributed to obesity?

10. According to current standards, how is obesity defined?

11. Briefly describe bulimia and identify the medical complications associated with it.

12. Compare and contrast substance abuse and substance dependence.

13. A substance abuser typically uses two key defense mechanisms—denial and isolation. Explain how these mechanisms prevent treatment and recovery.

14. What are the most common long-term effects of smoking?

15. Define alcoholism.

16. Describe the effects of alcohol consumption on individual health, the U.S. economy, and society.

17. What are some factors that cause particular stress for women?

18. A woman's responses to stress are shaped from birth. Socialization of women into traditional roles and responsibilities limits their options for learning new methods to cope with stress and change. Briefly describe the effects of negative socialization of women for each of the following four areas (identified by Griffith-Kenney): powerlessness, limited options, anger, and confusion of internal and external processes.

19. Identify at least six physiologic responses to stress.

20. Describe several nursing intervention strategies for each of the following health-compromising concerns: obesity, smoking, alcohol or drug abuse, and stress.

21. List the common signs and symptoms of abuse for each of the following drugs or drug classifications:
- amphetamines
- barbiturates
- cocaine
- hallucinogens
- marijuana
- opiates
- nicotine

Fill in the blank

22. Women and children make up more than ____________ of America's impoverished population.

23. Balancing multiple roles, such as holding a job, keeping house, and raising a family, may lead to improved self-esteem and ____________ for some women.

24. Because American women live longer than men, they are more likely to suffer the stresses of surviving a spouse, which include ____________ and ____________.

Matching terms and definitions

25. Match the appropriate description in the left column with each substance in the right column. (A description may apply to more than one substance.)

(1) substance obtained from the flowering tops, stems, and leaves of the hemp plant	(a) amphetamine
(2) central nervous system stimulant derived from coca leaves that causes euphoria and anesthetizes nerve endings	(b) barbituate
(3) synthetic narcotic used in detoxification programs to replace heroin	(c) cocaine
(4) sympathetic nervous system stimulant	(d) codeine
(5) addictive alkaloid found in tobacco; classified as a stimulant	(e) hallucinogen
(6) narcotic derived from opium; may relieve pain or induce sleep	(f) heroin
(7) nonnarcotic sedative that can cause physical and psychological dependence	(g) marijuana
(8) psychotomimetic drug that alters consciousness and causes hallucinations	(h) methadone
	(i) nicotine
	(j) morphine

Values clarification

To be an effective health care professional and role model for clients, the nurse should be aware of personal attitudes, feelings, and beliefs about good health. What do the following concepts of good health mean to you?

- self-actualization
- appropriate body image
- health life practices
- social involvement
- positive self-concept
- fitness
- full cognitive function
- positive mood
- harmony

Can you think of any other concepts to add to this list that express your definition of good health? How might your definition of good health affect your comfort level and professional competence in addressing your clients' health-compromising behaviors and concerns?

◆ CHAPTER 16 ◆

CONCEPTION AND FETAL DEVELOPMENT

CHAPTER OVERVIEW

In the months after an ovum is fertilized, cells divide and differentiate and intricate structures and systems form. A thorough knowledge of these processes is essential for the nurse who plans to teach, counsel, and provide anticipatory guidance to pregnant clients—or for the nurse who hopes to promote an optimal reproductive environment for clients planning conception. Chapter 16 provides the theoretical framework needed to fulfill these nursing roles. It describes gametogenesis and fertilization, identifying the various influences on these events. It examines prenatal development in three distinct phases: pre-embryonic, embryonic, and fetal development. Then it describes the components of the intrauterine environment, examining the circulation and endocrine functions of the placenta and describing the transfer of substances across the placenta.

STUDENT ACTIVITIES

To test your familiarity with the information in this chapter, complete the following activities.

Multiple choice

1. Which of the following developmental events does *not* take place during the pre-embryonic period? Explain your answer.
   (a) fertilization
   (b) implantation
   (c) cell division
   (d) formation of primitive organ systems

2. Which of the following gestational events occurs after the embryonic period ends? Explain your answer.
   (a) placental completion
   (b) development of organ systems
   (c) limb formation
   (d) ear and eye formation

3. Which of the following processes does *not* influence placental transfer?
   (a) facilitated diffusion
   (b) dialysis
   (c) active transport
   (d) pinocytosis

Study questions

4. Identify the four physiologic conditions that must be met before fertilization can occur.

5. Name the three germ layers that form specific tissues and organs within the embryo.

6. Briefly describe a gamete, a zygote, a morula, a blastocyst, and an embryo.

7. Which three embryonic structures unite to form the umbilical cord? When does this union typically take place?

8. Describe the two major events of the embryonic period, and explain their nursing implications.

9. Identify the approximate week(s) of gestation during which each of the following events occurs:
(a) The lungs produce surfactant to prepare for a functioning respiratory system.
(b) The kidneys begin to function and secrete urine.
(c) Vernix covers the skin to protect against the drying action of amniotic fluid.
(d) The fetus is considered viable.
(e) Myelination of the brain begins.
(f) The placenta is complete and fetal circulation has developed.
(g) Sucking and swallowing occur.
(h) Muscle movements are detectable.
(i) Meconium is present in the bowel.
(j) The brain is grossly formed.

10. Describe the functions of amniotic fluid, the process of amniotic fluid production, and the circulation of amniotic fluid during gestation.

11. What are the three major functions of the placenta during the gestational period?

12. Briefly describe the three shunts that permit the fetal circulation to bypass the liver and lungs.

Fill in the blank

13. The ____________ is the germ layer that forms the embryo's external covering as well as the organs contacting the environment.

14. The middle germ layer, which forms supporting tissues and other structures, is called the ____________ .

15. The ____________ is the embryo's internal lining.

◆ CHAPTER 17 ◆

PHYSIOLOGIC CHANGES DURING NORMAL PREGNANCY

CHAPTER OVERVIEW

During pregnancy, the body undergoes wide-ranging changes to help maintain overall health, create a nurturing environment for the fetus, and prepare for labor and delivery. To promote the health of the pregnant client more effectively, the nurse must have a thorough understanding of these changes. Chapter 17 provides the conceptual basis the nurse requires. It discusses the presumptive, probable, and positive signs of pregnancy; describes the physiologic changes occurring in all major body systems; and explains the hormonal influences that initiate or regulate body functions during pregnancy. To help the nurse provide accurate information and nursing care for the pregnant client, the chapter also discusses the signs and symptoms resulting from these changes.

STUDENT ACTIVITIES

To test your familiarity with the information in this chapter, complete the following activities.

Clinical simulations

1. Phyllis, age 31, comes to the health center for a pregnancy test, stating that she has not had a menstrual period for 3 months. She feels sure she is pregnant because, she says, "I've never missed a period until now." She and her husband have been trying to conceive for over a year. Should the nurse regard Phyllis' amenorrhea as a presumptive, probable, or positive sign of pregnancy? Explain your answer.

2. Phyllis also reports nausea and vomiting, abdominal enlargement, breast changes, and fatigue. Of these signs and symptoms, which one is a probable sign of pregnancy? Explain your answer.

3. Liz Martino, a 25-year-old primigravid client at 36 weeks' gestation, reports that a sticky yellow substance has been leaking from her nipples for several weeks. She asks, "Isn't it too soon for breast milk to come in?" How should the nurse explain these breast secretions and the changes that Liz should anticipate?

4. Eighteen weeks into her pregnancy, Karen, a primigravid client age 28, comes to the clinic complaining of a "constantly stuffy nose" and a recent episode of epistaxis. How should the nurse explain the causes of these typical pregnancy-related changes?

5. Dianne, age 31, visits the prenatal clinic at 28 weeks' gestation complaining of chronic heartburn. What condition should the nurse suspect as the cause of her complaint?

6. Renata Stephenson, a nurse educator, is planning to discuss prenatal cervical changes in her childbirth education class. How would she describe the mucus plug?

7. During a subsequent childbirth education class, Jim Hunter, an expectant father, tells Renata Stephenson that his wife Arlene has chronic backache and that her expanding abdomen is affecting the way she walks and stands. Several other men in the class say they have seen similar changes in their partners. What explanation should Renata provide for these changes?

8. Marta, a primigravid client age 28, is 16 weeks' pregnant when she makes a routine visit to the prenatal clinic. During the nursing assessment, she asks if something is wrong with her pregnancy because she looks so much smaller than her friend Angela, who is 16 weeks into her fourth pregnancy. What should the nurse tell her?

9. Betty Greenfeld, a primigravid client who is 32 weeks pregnant, tells the nurse she is upset about the striae gravidarum (stretch marks) on her abdomen and breasts. She asks the nurse what causes them and whether they will be permanent. What should the nurse tell her?

10. Olga Resevich, 33 weeks pregnant, comes to the clinic for an unscheduled prenatal visit because she has been experiencing a "strange numbness" on her thigh. The physician diagnoses meralgia paresthetica. Describe this neurologic condition of pregnancy.

Study questions

11. Name two positive signs of pregnancy and state how they are identified.

12. Morning sickness (nausea and vomiting) is common during the first trimester of pregnancy. When is this condition considered abnormal?

13. Describe the effects of increased blood volume during pregnancy and the early postpartal period.

14. Which anatomic changes predispose the pregnant client to urinary tract infection?

15. How does the funic souffle differ from the uterine souffle?

16. Identify and describe skin changes occurring during pregnancy.

17. What does the term "quickening" mean?

Fill in the blank

18. During pregnancy, vaginal secretions normally ____________.

19. The posterior pituitary gland releases vasopressin and oxytocin during pregnancy. Vasopressin helps regulate water balance through its ____________ action; oxytocin stimulates labor and aids in ____________ through its effect on breast tissue.

20. The placenta secretes a hormone called human placental lactogen, which promotes breakdown of ____________ and provides an alternate source of energy.

21. In response to hormonal changes, the respiratory system undergoes both biochemical changes and ____________ changes during pregnancy.

22. Alterations in blood volume, cardiac output, and heart size and position cause changes in heart ____________ during pregnancy.

True or false

23. Vasodilation and heat intolerance during pregnancy reflect endocrine dysfunction.
❑ True ❑ False

24. Pregnancy alters the cardiovascular system so profoundly that the resulting changes would be considered pathologic in a nonpregnant client.
❑ True ❑ False

25. Systolic and diastolic blood pressures decrease from hormonal influences during pregnancy, especially in the last half of the second trimester.
❑ True ❑ False

26. Brachial artery pressure is highest when the pregnant client lies on her back.
❑ True ❑ False

27. Because the developing fetus requires increasing calcium and phosphorus, the incidence of dental caries increases during pregnancy.
❑ True ❑ False

28. During pregnancy, liver function studies typically show changes that would suggest hepatic disease in a nonpregnant woman.
❑ True ❑ False

29. Sodium requirements increase during pregnancy because the client needs more intravascular and extracellular fluid.
❑ True ❑ False

Matching terms and definitions

30. Match each probable sign of pregnancy in the left column with the appropriate description in the right column.

(1) Braun von Fernwald's sign	(a) bluish coloration of the mucous membranes of the cervix, vagina, and vulva
(2) Chadwick's sign	(b) easy flexion of the fundus into the cervix
(3) Goodell's sign	(c) softening of the cervix
(4) Hegar's sign	(d) softening of the uterine isthmus
(5) Ladin's sign	(e) fullness and irregular softness of the fundus near the area of implantation
(6) McDonald's sign	(f) soft, palpable area on the anterior middle portion of the uterus near the junction of the uterus and cervix

◆ CHAPTER 18 ◆

PSYCHOSOCIAL CHANGES DURING NORMAL PREGNANCY

CHAPTER OVERVIEW

Profound psychosocial changes accompany the dramatic physiologic alterations of pregnancy. The transition to parenthood brings changes in responsibilities, life-styles, values, relationships, and self-image. To prepare the nurse to promote an optimal psychosocial adjustment to childbearing, Chapter 18 explores these issues. It discusses the factors that affect a couple's transition to parenthood and describes the emotional and social tasks of the expectant mother and father during each trimester. After investigating the effects of pregnancy on the couple's relationship and on their successful adaptation to childbearing, it discusses preparation of the siblings and grandparents for the arrival of a new family member. The chapter also describes the cultural and family variations that may affect a family's experience of pregnancy and childbirth.

STUDENT ACTIVITIES

To test your familiarity with the information in this chapter, complete the following activities.

Clinical simulations

1. Sonia, age 29, is pregnant with her second child. At 9 weeks' gestation, she visits her obstetrician to seek help for persistent morning sickness. She and her husband Alan, age 31, have just relocated from Germany, where Alan was stationed for military duty. Once he completes his 2-month assignment here, he expects to be reassigned; the uncertainty over this situation has placed a strain on both their marriage and budget. While awaiting Alan's reassignment, the couple and their son Nathaniel, age 11 months, are living with Sonia's parents. Identify at least four sources of stress for Sonia and Alan during this pregnancy.

2. Which two conscious or unconscious mechanisms might Sonia use in response to the increased stress and uncertainty she is facing?

3. During the history interview, Sonia makes the statements shown below. Which statement reflects her use of a coping mechanism rather than a defense mechanism? Explain your answer.
   (a) "I just don't think about my problems."
   (b) "All I do is think about how nice and simple our life was back on the base in Germany."

(c) "My family has been very helpful in preparing us for our next move."
(d) "I sleep all the time to forget my problems."

4. Identify at least five suggestions the nurse could make to help Sonia cope with her problems more effectively.

5. Peter and his wife Judy are expecting their first child in less than 1 month. Devoted to Judy throughout her pregnancy, Peter has been anticipating the birth of their child with great excitement, accompanying Judy on each prenatal visit. During a routine visit at 37 weeks' gestation, he confides to the nurse that he feels as if he is pregnant, too, because of his nausea, chronic low backache, restlessness at night, inability to concentrate at work, and increased irritability. Judy teasingly adds that he has gained almost as much weight as she has during her pregnancy.
How should the nurse explain Peter's signs and symptoms to the couple?

6. During a prenatal visit at 28 weeks' gestation, Damita reports that her dreams have been more intense since she became pregnant. She recounts a strange dream she had the previous night, in which she lost her baby in a shopping mall; she looked everywhere but could not find the baby, and woke up frantic. She asks the nurse why she keeps having strange dreams and what the dreams might mean. How should the nurse reply?

7. Describe how the nurse could help Damita to interpret her dream about the lost baby and thus promote her conflict resolution.

8. During a childbirth preparation class, the nurse educator asks the couples to brainstorm about the psychosocial tasks they currently face. The women are in their third trimester; most are due to deliver in about 6 weeks. The nurse educator should expect these couples to identify which psychosocial tasks?

9. Renee and her husband Joe have chosen to have their sons, ages 4 and 6, attend the birth of their third child. Renee asks the nurse how she and Joe can help prepare the boys for the childbirth to make it a more positive experience for them. Identify some appropriate suggestions the nurse could make.

Multiple choice

10. The first trimester of pregnancy is known as the trimester of:
(a) adaptation
(b) ambivalence
(c) prenatal attachment
(d) preparation for parenting

11. What is the main psychological task of an expectant father during the first trimester?
(a) to develop his father image
(b) to begin paternal-fetal attachment
(c) to choose his level of involvement with the pregnancy
(d) to accept the reality of the pregnancy

Study questions

12. What makes childbearing a unique experience for the family?

13. To help the expectant family adapt to and integrate a new family member, the nurse must address which five major psychosocial goals?

14. Explain how a nurse working with pregnant clients can promote the client's right to self-determination.

15. Describe one way in which the nurse can help meet the psychosocial needs of the expectant family in each of the following settings: the health care facility, the community, and society.

16. What role do coping mechanisms play in solving problems?

17. Briefly define defense mechanisms, and explain how a person might use them to deal with a problem.

18. List four aspects of the mother-daughter relationship that influence a woman's mother image.

19. Which aspects of the prospective father's life influence his role development during the second trimester of pregnancy?

20. During the second trimester, a client typically demonstrates which attachment behaviors toward her fetus?

21. Describe common changes in body image and sexuality during the second trimester.

22. Why do some parents choose to have their children present during birth?

23. What role do grandparents play within the family?

True or false

24. A child's display of jealousy toward a new sibling usually indicates that the child feels unloved.
❑ True ❑ False

25. A woman who has prepared herself realistically will not experience anxiety about labor and delivery.
❑ True ❑ False

26. For a client who values the childbirth experience, self-esteem may be linked to her performance during labor and delivery.
❑ True ❑ False

27. Death is such an irrational fear during childbirth that clients rarely express this concern.
❑ True ❑ False

28. Studies of married couples show that the wife's adjustment to or enjoyment of pregnancy does not increase when the husband receives emotional support.
❑ True ❑ False

29. The way a pregnant client and her partner view her body changes will affect her sexual responsiveness and self-image.
❑ True ❑ False

◆ CHAPTER 19 ◆

CARE DURING THE NORMAL ANTEPARTAL PERIOD

CHAPTER OVERVIEW

Antepartal nursing care aims to promote and maintain the health and well-being of the client and fetus throughout pregnancy. The nurse caring for the pregnant client must be able to recognize the signs of a healthy, progressive pregnancy; assess for common discomforts of pregnancy; identify antepartal risk factors promptly so that appropriate interventions can begin; and provide appropriate teaching and counseling. Chapter 19 provides the foundation for the nurse to fulfill these roles. It describes the components of antepartal assessment, discusses the normal physiologic changes of pregnancy during each trimester, and describes the physical examination conducted to detect such changes. It explains how to promote client and family adaptation to pregnancy and minimize antepartal risks and discomfort. The chapter elaborates on antepartal client-teaching topics and reviews the items to evaluate and document when providing nursing care for the pregnant client.

STUDENT ACTIVITIES

To test your familiarity with the information in this chapter, complete the following activities.

Clinical simulations

1. Sondra is 6 weeks pregnant, based on the dates of her last menstrual period (LMP). During the prenatal history interview, she tells the nurse that she has had three children by vaginal delivery at term, one preterm neonate who died shortly after birth at 26 weeks' gestation, and two abortions at about 8 weeks' gestation. Of the following, which is the correct way to document Sondra's previous pregnancies, using the TPAL system? Explain your answer.
   (a) gravida 6, para 3213
   (b) gravida 7, para 4024
   (c) gravida 7, para 3123
   (d) gravida 7, para 3024

2. The first day of Sondra's LMP was January 7. She has regular menstrual cycles and was not using contraception when she conceived. Using Nagele's rule, calculate her expected date of delivery (EDD).

3. Terry Mason comes to the clinic for a routine prenatal examination at 24 weeks' gestation. Her pregnancy has been uneventful; her measured fundal height consistently has equaled gestational age in

weeks. Assuming that this pattern still holds, the nurse practitioner expect to measure what fundal height during this visit?

4. Nina, a 25-year-old gravida 2, para 1001 client who is 30 weeks pregnant, seems distracted during a routine prenatal visit. She tells the nurse that her daughter Kristine, age 3, has seemed frustrated and aggressive when playing with her dolls since learning of Nina's pregnancy. She fears Kristine will have problems adjusting to a sibling. How can the nurse help Nina deal with Kristine's behavior and feelings?

5. Josie arrives at the nurse-midwife's office for a regular prenatal examination. A gravida 3, para 2002 client at 28 weeks' gestation, she complains of a chronic backache—especially after a long day of caring for her rambunctious daughter, age 18 months, and son, age 3. After determining that Josie's backache is a normal discomfort of pregnancy rather than a sign of a more serious problem, the nurse-midwife might suggest which comfort measures?

6. Pat Stoddard, age 17, is a primigravid client who complains of constipation during a prenatal examination. Describe at least four measures the nurse might recommend to improve Pat's bowel elimination pattern.

Study questions

7. List three methods for predicting the EDD when the client cannot remember the date of her LMP or has irregular menses.

8. A client should be assessed how frequently during the antepartal period?

9. List the seven major components of a health history that the nurse should collect during the initial assessment of a pregnant client.

10. Provide an appropriate response to each of the following questions commonly asked by clients during early prenatal visits.
(a) When will I be able to hear my baby's heartbeat?
(b) When will I be able to feel the baby kicking?
(c) How soon will my pregnancy show? (Assume the client is pregnant for the first time.)

11. How does the nurse determine fetal status when assessing a pregnant client?

12. List the laboratory tests that are performed routinely on pregnant clients.

13. The nurse should cover which general categories when teaching a client about antepartal care measures that enhance client and fetal well-being?

14. Identify the danger signs that the nurse should review with clients during each routine prenatal visit.

15. Describe some ways in which pregnant clients can assess fetal well-being by monitoring movement.

16. Which factors can alter fetal activity?

◆ CHAPTER 20 ◆

NUTRITION AND DIET COUNSELING

CHAPTER OVERVIEW

Preconception and antepartal nutrition play a key role in the course and outcome of pregnancy. To promote and maintain the health of the pregnant client and her fetus, the nurse must address the client's nutritional concerns. The nurse teaches about proper nutrition and its importance to the developing fetus, stays alert for signs of nutritional problems or adverse personal habits that could harm the client's or fetus's well-being, and implements appropriate intervention strategies. Chapter 20 examines the nutritional requirements of the pregnant client and explores nutrition-related factors that may affect pregnancy outcome. It reviews the roles of specific nutrients during pregnancy, describing their influence on nutritional status, and explores antepartal nutritional risk factors. Then the chapter presents nutrition-related nursing care to promote an optimal pregnancy outcome, elaborating on client teaching.

STUDENT ACTIVITIES

To test your familiarity with the information in this chapter, complete the following activities.

Clinical simulations

1. Eighteen weeks pregnant, Angela Riccone, a single, 20-year-old, unemployed mother of three, comes to the health clinic for an initial prenatal examination. The nursing health history reveals that Angela delivered her first child at age 16 and that her children were born 1 to 2 years apart; she was treated for anemia during her previous pregnancies, and she smokes one pack of cigarettes daily. Physical examination finds Angela thin and pale, with a fundal height that measures small for gestational age. Preliminary laboratory studies reveal severe anemia. Based on these findings, the nurse determines that Angela is at high risk for malnutrition and refers her to the Special Supplemental Food Program for Women, Infants and Children (WIC). Explain how this program can help Angela improve her pregnancy outcome and enhance her family's nutritional status.

2. During a prenatal nutrition class for pregnant adolescents, the nurse educator explains that the average pregnant adult in her ideal weight range should gain a total of 24 to 32 pounds—but that an adolescent may need to gain additional weight depending on her stage of growth and development. Morgan, a 15-year-old primigravid client, tells the class, "I'm not going to gain that much weight. I don't want to look like a blimp." Morgan is in her second year after menarche and is slightly underweight. How should the nurse educator respond to her comment?

3. Lilia, age 36, recently immigrated to the United States from Guatemala. She has delivered two full-term neonates and two premature neonates, has had four miscarriages, and has three living children. She and her husband are migrant farm workers who live below the poverty level despite their long hours of work in the fields. Lilia is obese, and she reports that her diet consists mainly of rice, beans, and plantains. She is under close observation for hypertension, for which she takes medication. Explain why Lilia would be at nutritional risk should she become pregnant again.

4. Georgia Kreger, age 38, is obese. Twenty-four weeks into her third pregnancy, a routine fasting 1-hour glucose tolerance test (GTT) and a follow-up 3-hour GTT reveal that she has gestational diabetes. When counseling Georgia about prenatal nutrition, the nurse should emphasize which principles?

5. Dawn Caldwell, 20 weeks pregnant, is diagnosed with iron-deficiency anemia. List at least five suggestions the nurse could make to help enhance her dietary iron intake.

6. Roberta, a 24-year-old primigravid client, arrives for her initial prenatal visit at 8 weeks' gestation. She has a history of lactose intolerance and states that she cannot eat dairy products. To increase Roberta's calcium intake, the nurse should recommend how much calcium supplementation and should suggest which other dietary measures?

7. Julie and her husband George are vegans—they consume no animal products. During a routine prenatal home visit, the public health nurse discusses alternative ways to ensure that Julie, now 12 weeks pregnant, consumes adequate, complete proteins and calories in her daily diet. Describe one meal plan that the nurse might recommend.

8. Carmen, age 20, is a primigravid client who is 16 weeks pregnant when she arrives for her initial prenatal visit. By her report, she has gained 20 pounds during her pregnancy. During a dietary recall, she provides the following information about her intake on the day before this visit:
8 a.m.: two bowls of corn flakes with milk and sugar, one scrambled egg, a glass of orange juice, a glass of milk
11 a.m.: a slice of bread with butter, coffee with cream and 2 tsp. sugar
12:30 p.m.: homemade chicken-vegetable soup, rice, plantains, pudding, soft drink 4 p.m.: two pastries, coffee with cream and 2 tsp. sugar
6 p.m.: baked chicken with rice and beans, water, ice cream
9 pm: one orange, some cookies, water.
Based on this information, fill out the diet table on the following page. Then identify the deficiencies and excesses in Carmen's diet, and provide appropriate nursing recommendations to help Carmen make better food choices.

Carmen's food plan table

	Protein	Dairy	Fruit/vegetable	Bread/cereal	Sugar/fat	Fluid
Recommended servings	3	4	4	4	0	8 glasses
Carmen's diet						

Multiple choice

9. A well-nourished pregnant client must consume how many extra calories daily during the second and third trimesters to meet the increased needs of pregnancy?
(a) 150
(b) 350
(c) 500
(d) 800

10. Which two fat-soluble vitamins can cause fetal toxicity if ingested in excess of the recommended doses?
(a) vitamins A and D
(b) vitamins C and B_{12}
(c) vitamins B_6 and K
(d) vitamins B_1 (riboflavin) and E

Study questions

11. Which preconception factors can influence nutrition and pregnancy outcome?

12. Describe the pattern of expected weight gain during each trimester for a single-fetus pregnancy. Explain how this differs from the weight-gain pattern during a twin-fetus pregnancy.

13. Identify the six essential nutrients, and discuss their basic functions in health maintenance.

14. Describe the two primary methods of evaluating the nutritional intake of a pregnant client, and state the advantages and disadvantages of each method.

15. To maintain a balanced diet, the pregnant client should consume how many daily servings from each of the four basic food groups?

16. Which factors may influence a client's food choices and should be taken into consideration by the nurse when developing a meal plan?

17. A client should drink approximately how much fluid each day to meet the demands of pregnancy?

◆ CHAPTER 21 ◆

FAMILY PREPARATION FOR CHILDBIRTH AND PARENTING

CHAPTER OVERVIEW

During the past few decades, consumerism and greater family participation in health care have increased the demand for childbirth and parenting education. Such education has become more complex and sophisticated; childbearing and child-rearing families now can choose from a wide range of educational options. Classes are available not just for expectant parents but also for siblings, grandparents, friends, and others with an interest in the expectant family. Many sources offer childbirth and parenting education, including health care facilities, national organizations, independent educators, and consumer-based community organizations. With so many opportunities to teach expectant families, the nurse must be knowledgeable about childbirth techniques, childbirth preparation methods, trends in maternal-child health care, and ways to help the expectant client and her partner make a healthy transition to parenthood. Chapter 21 reviews the roles and responsibilities of the nurse as childbirth educator. Besides discussing adult learning principles and the common components of childbirth education classes, it describes nurse educator roles, explains how to recognize role conflicts associated with parenting, and reviews educational techniques that promote role transition for expectant couples. The chapter also summarizes childbirth preparation methods.

STUDENT ACTIVITIES

To test your familiarity with the information in this chapter, complete the following activities.

Clinical simulations

1. Ina Rogers, a nurse in the new family-centered maternity wing at Memorial Hospital, is developing a childbirth preparation and parenting course for expectant families in the local community. Before deciding which topics to include in the course, she must formulate overall educational goals that reflect the general purpose of the course. Identify five overall goals that Ina likely will develop.

2. Based on the overall educational goals Ina has formulated, she decides that her course will incorporate 14 topics. Identify the educational goal or goals shown in the left column that each topic in the right column meets. (A topic may meet more than one goal.)

(1) making informed choices	(a) pain management interventions: analgesia and anesthesia
(2) ensuring antepartal health	(b) natural labor and childbirth
(3) coping with pregnancy, labor, and childbirth	(c) eating for two during pregnancy
(4) dealing with infant care	(d) progressive relaxation and breathing techniques during labor
(5) making the transition to parenthood	(e) neonatal care
	(f) serving as family advocate: communicating with health care professionals
	(g) childbirth satisfaction through goal-setting
	(h) postpartal adjustment
	(i) preparing for the unexpected childbirth experience
	(j) sibling preparation for childbirth
	(k) prenatal health maintenance strategies
	(l) balancing children and careers
	(m) vaginal birth after cesarean delivery: what to expect
	(n) reproductive and contraceptive alternatives

3. Which educational goal is common to all of the topics Ina will incorporate into her course? What information must Ina provide in her course to meet this goal?

4. Lynne, a new graduate nurse, believes women should learn to be advocates for the health and well-being of their families. She had positive childbirth experiences of her own by using prepared childbirth techniques; as a nursing student, she enjoyed teaching clients. Now that Lynne works in a private obstetrics practice, she would like to become involved in childbirth education. Besides teaching clients during routine prenatal visits, which educator roles would allow Lynne to meet her clients' teaching needs? For each educator role,

describe Lynne's responsibilities and identify the additional preparation she would need.

5. Joyce Sinkowski, a nurse educator, is preparing a prenatal education course for inner city women with marginal literacy. To tailor her course to these students, which learning characteristics must Joyce keep in mind?

Study questions

6. Define the purpose of childbirth education.

7. To determine the informational needs of the childbearing family, the nurse must assess which areas?

8. Identify six components that commonly are incorporated into every childbirth education course.

9. Provide a detailed description of the patterned paced breathing technique, using terms a nurse educator would use when teaching this technique to a childbirth preparation class.

10. Describe the pelvic tilt-on-all-fours exercise.

11. Why should a childbirth education course include a discussion of the transition to parenthood?

12. According to Rubin, four specific tasks prepare the expectant client for the maternal role. List these tasks.

13. When teaching expectant couples, the nurse educator must address role conflicts to ensure a successful transition to parenthood. Identify at least three issues that can lead to role conflicts for expectant mothers; do the same for expectant fathers.

Matching terms and definitions

14. To assess the learning characteristics of individual clients in a childbirth education class, the nurse educator might analyze the statements they make. Match each client statement, shown in the left column, with the specific characteristic of adult learners, shown in the right column, that best reflects the client's learning style.

(1) "I read in a professional journal that vaginal birth after cesarean delivery is safe for the mother and baby in certain circumstances. The statistics were reassuring. What is your opinion?"	(a) is interested in immediate application of knowledge
(2) "My wife and I have gone through childbirth before. This time, we want to learn and understand more about the effects of relaxation technique during labor."	(b) values participation in learning

(3) "I used my modified paced breathing and relaxation techniques at the dentist's last week, and found that it really made a difference."

(4) "My husband and I talked with our son last week to help prepare him for his new baby brother or sister. How should we handle the homecoming from the hospital so that it's a positive experience for him?"

(5) "I find labor-rehearsal role-playing helpful because it gives me some concrete ideas of what to expect before I have to cope with the real thing."

(c) has a self-directed learning style

(d) values learning that facilitates mastery of current developmental tasks or is problem-focused and relevant to the situation

(e) has a background of previous experiences that may facilitate learning

15. Every childbirth preparation method reflects a distinct philosophy. Match each method shown in the left column with the corresponding philosophy in the right column.

(1) Dick-Read's childbirth without fear method

(2) Lamaze, or psychoprophylactic, method

(3) Bradley's husband-coached childbirth method

(4) Kitzinger's psychosexual method

(a) Birth is a natural occurrence; the client's husband is the best person to support her during labor because he is involved fully in all aspects of the pregnancy and childbirth.

(b) Women can be self-reliant during childbirth because they have an instinct for and innate knowledge of the process. Childbirth is a sexual experience that should be experienced with spontaneity and freedom.

(c) The client focuses on internal sensory experiences so that she can respond to her body signals. Body awareness enhances the sensuality of childbirth, which is similar to orgasm.

(d) Active mental and physical conditioning and a controlled birth experience are crucial. Relaxation and breathing exercises promote mental control over pain. Through conditioned response techniques, the client learns to respond to pain with breathing and relaxation.

(5) LeBoyer's birth-without-violence method	(e) Labor is a normal physiologic process in which the client should maintain awareness of body feelings and rely on her ability to cope with labor.
(6) Noble's gentle pushing method	(f) Knowledge about childbirth can break the fear-tension-pain cycle of childbirth and allow a natural childbirth. Anesthesia and analgesics should be avoided.
(7) Odent's instinctive birth method	(g) The external environment surrounding the birth is important to neonatal adaptation. Use of soft lights, gentle music, and a warm, comforting environment eases the neonate's transition to the extrauterine environment.

Values clarification

The nurse educator's philosophy of childbirth education and presentation of course material are influenced by personal attitudes, feelings, and beliefs. To help assess your attitudes, feelings, and beliefs about childbirth and childbirth education, complete each of the following sentences with the first thought that comes to mind. (You may find this exercise more meaningful after completing Unit 4 of the text. However, you may use it now to guide your developing philosophy of childbirth.)

16. When I think about childbirth as a natural process, I ...

17. To promote health maintenance during pregnancy, effective prenatal teaching should include ...

18. I believe that modern technology and intervention in obstetrics are ...

19. When I hear someone say that a woman should have total control over her childbirth experience, I feel...

20. A childbirth educator who influences the expectations and decisions of a prenatal couple by directing their choice of childbirth goals is...

21. The most effective way to improve birthing practices and options in my community is to ...

22. If the policies of a health care facility do not support a couple's goals for their childbirth experience, I would advise them to ...

23. I believe the need for medication in labor is ...

24. Informed choices in childbirth mean ...

25. When it comes to teaching about unexpected complications of childbirth, I would ...

What did you just discover about your attitudes, feelings, and beliefs about childbirth? How might these attitudes, feelings, and beliefs affect your philosophy of childbirth education and your presentation of course material?

◆ CHAPTER 22 ◆

HIGH-RISK ANTEPARTAL CLIENTS

CHAPTER OVERVIEW

Certain medical problems, age-related concerns, and socioeconomic factors can result in a high-risk pregnancy that jeopardizes maternal or fetal health or impedes normal fetal development, childbirth, or the transition to parenthood. Nursing care for the high-risk antepartal client and her family aims to provide optimal prenatal care and promote safe delivery of a neonate in peak health. Chapter 22 explores the conditions that lead to a high-risk pregnancy. It discusses the physical and social risks faced by adolescent and mature antepartal clients, examines the implications of selected medical problems on pregnancy, and outlines the special management needs of the pregnant client who suffers trauma or requires surgery. Then the chapter outlines nursing care for the high-risk antepartal client, describing both invasive and noninvasive fetal tests that may be ordered as well as the health monitoring and teaching the client requires. It also presents appropriate nursing measures, such as those that promote client rest, exercise, nutrition, and compliance.

STUDENT ACTIVITIES

To test your familiarity with the information in this chapter, complete the following activities.

Clinical simulations

1. Heather Austin, a high school freshman age 14, is referred to the prenatal clinic by her family physician after a routine school physical examination reveals she is 33 weeks pregnant. (Her baggy clothing has hidden her condition from her parents and teachers.) Explain why Heather is at risk during this pregnancy, and identify some of the risks she and her neonate face.

2. Describe some ways in which the nurse at Heather's prenatal clinic can foster a healthier outcome for her and her fetus at this time in her pregnancy.

3. Mary DeSanto, a primigravid client age 39, is about to undergo amniocentesis to investigate the possibility of fetal chromosomal abnormalities associated with her age. When teaching Mary and her husband about this procedure, the nurse should provide what information?

4. Helen Foster, age 40, was 26 weeks pregnant when diagnosed with gestational diabetes mellitus. Since then, she has been monitored closely; her blood glucose levels have remained stable because of her careful adherence to a proper diet. Results of initial genetic testing (for age-related concerns) were normal, and Helen has re-

mained in good general health. As Helen enters week 36 of pregnancy, the nurse should anticipate that the physician will order which fetal evaluation tests?

5. Ruby Davis, age 32, comes to the health clinic for a routine prenatal visit at 24 weeks' gestation. She complains of headaches, pallor, chronic fatigue and weakness, and exertional dyspnea. She also reports symptoms of anorexia—although confessing to a craving for laundry starch—and says she has been unusually irritable with her husband and children. When questioned, she admits she often forgets to take her iron and vitamin supplements. The nurse should suspect which disorder as the cause of Ruby's complaints? Which tests typically are ordered to diagnose this disorder?

6. Describe the potential risks to Ruby and her fetus or neonate if her disorder remains untreated.

7. What is the recommended treatment for Ruby's disorder? When teaching Ruby about her disorder and its treatment, the nurse should include which topics?

8. Jill Lafferty, age 32, is 36 weeks pregnant. When she arrives for a routine prenatal visit smelling of alcohol and speaking in a slurred manner, the nurse asks if she has been drinking. She admits she takes a drink "every now and then." On further questioning, the nurse determines that Jill consumes three to four beers on two to three occasions every week and occasionally drinks a six-pack of beer if she is under unusual stress. How should the nurse proceed?

Multiple choice

9. Which of the following measures is *not* part of the treatment regimen for a pregnant diabetic client? Explain your answer.
(a) dietary changes
(b) home glucose monitoring
(c) bed rest
(d) insulin administration

10. Which of the following is *not* a neonatal effect of heavy cigarette smoking (nicotine abuse) during pregnancy?
(a) an increased risk for sudden infant death syndrome
(b) small-for-gestational-age status
(c) intrauterine hypoxia (decreased placental perfusion)
(d) chromosomal damage

Study questions

11. Identify five common surgical procedures performed on pregnant clients.

12. A biophysical profile (BPP) evaluates fetal health by assessing specific variables. Describe the purposes of a BPP and identify the specific variables it assesses.

13. Compare and contrast the results of the non-stress test (NST) and n ipple stimulation contraction stress test used to assess fetal well-being.

14. Explain the meaning of the term TORCH, and discuss the clinical significance of TORCH infections during pregnancy.

15. What are two primary causes of trauma during pregnancy?

16. When is a sickle cell crisis most likely to occur in pregnant clients with sickle cell disease?

17. How does diabetes mellitus affect the pregnant client?

18. What is the prognosis for a pregnant client with rheumatic heart disease?

19. Describe general management guidelines for the pregnant client with cardiac disease.

True or false

20. During the third trimester, the normal physiologic changes of pregnancy decrease stress on the heart.
❑ True ❑ False

21. Rheumatic heart disease is the most common cardiac disorder among pregnant clients.
❑ True ❑ False

22. All pregnant clients should be screened for glucose intolerance with a 1-hour (50-gram) diabetes screening test.
❑ True ❑ False

23. The neonate of a client with advanced diabetes mellitus may show signs of intrauterine growth retardation.
❑ True ❑ False

24. Congenital anomalies are not associated with maternal insulin-dependent diabetes mellitus.
❑ True ❑ False

25. If a neonate who was delivered through a birth canal infected with herpesvirus initially lacks signs and symptoms of herpes, no cause for alarm exists.
❑ True ❑ False

26. The fetus of a woman who carries the human immunodeficiency virus may not necessarily contract the disease.
❑ True ❑ False

27. If a pregnant client with trichomoniasis does not receive prompt treatment, her neonate is at risk for contracting ophthalmia neonatorum during vaginal delivery.
❑ True ❑ False

28. Maternal cocaine use can cause fetal chromosomal abnormalities, resulting in major genitourinary malformations.
❑ True ❑ False

◆ CHAPTER 23 ◆

ANTEPARTAL COMPLICATIONS

CHAPTER OVERVIEW

A medical or obstetric complication that threatens a pregnancy causes a crisis for the client and her family: As they alter their expectations about the future, they may feel fear and anxiety; as they try to understand why the complication occurred, they may experience guilt or blame. Chapter 23 prepares the nurse to care for the client with an antepartal complication, describing how to meet the psychosocial needs of both the client and her family while safeguarding the client's health. The chapter begins by examining the reproductive system disorders that may complicate pregnancy, discussing the etiology and incidence of such problems as spontaneous abortion, ectopic pregnancy, gestational trophoblastic disease, incompetent cervix, premature rupture of the membranes (PROM), and preterm labor and delivery. Then it focuses on antepartal complications arising from multisystemic disorders—hyperemesis gravidarum, hypertensive disorders, and Rh incompatibility. Describing nursing care, it identifies the history and physical findings that help assess each complication and offers nursing interventions to promote the client's well-being, prevent or control further complications or sequelae, and provide emotional support.

STUDENT ACTIVITIES

To test your familiarity with the information in this chapter, complete the following activities.

Clinical simulations

1. Stephanie Francis, a 26-year-old gravida 2, para 0010 client, is 6 weeks pregnant, based on the date of her last menstrual period (LMP). When confirming her pregnancy on her first prenatal visit, the physician assures her that everything is proceeding on schedule. One week later, however, Stephanie calls the prenatal clinic to report vaginal bleeding. The bleeding makes Stephanie particularly anxious because she had a miscarriage at the same stage in her first pregnancy last year. When the nurse questions her further, Stephanie states that she does not have cramps; the bleeding, which she noticed on the tissue paper after voiding, is scant and mixed with mucus. The nurse's suspicions center on the two most common causes of bleeding during the first trimester. Identify these causes, and describe how the nurse should proceed.

2. When Stephanie arrives for medical evaluation, the physician performs a speculum examination, which reveals a closed cervix and a uterine size compatible with her LMP. Based on the history and physical findings, the physician determines that Stephanie is experiencing a threatened abortion. The nurse should expect the physi-

cian to prescribe which measures for Stephanie? The nurse should provide what guidance for her?

3. Delores Ross, a primigravid client age 38, is pregnant with twins after undergoing successful clomiphene citrate therapy for infertility. During a routine prenatal examination at 28 weeks' gestation, the nurse measures her blood pressure at 140/96 mm Hg. Delores reports a past medical history of labile hypertension. Explain why the nurse suspects that Delores is developing pregnancy-induced hypertension (PIH).

4. The nurse should assess Delores for which other signs and symptoms to help the physician confirm a diagnosis of PIH?

5. The physician orders careful antepartal home monitoring for Delores. However, at 32 weeks' gestation, she is admitted to the labor and delivery area with a diagnosis of severe preeclampsia. What are four nursing goals for her care at this time?

6. Karline Kilgallen is a single primigravid client age 17, who dropped out of high school last year to work so she could help her mother support her six siblings. On her initial prenatal examination, the nurse measures her weight at 92 lb and her height at 5′. Karline states that she smokes a pack and a half of cigarettes at her job on an assembly line; she recalls being hospitalized for a kidney infection at age 13. Which factors in Karline's history point to the need for increased antepartal surveillance for preterm labor?

7. At 27 weeks' gestation, Karline is hospitalized for an episode of preterm labor. Her discharge plan includes an in-home uterine monitoring program. When preparing Karline for discharge, how should the nurse teach her about this program?

8. Barbara Chernow, a primigravid client age 32 who is 9 weeks pregnant, comes to the emergency department complaining of sudden abdominal pain. She reports that the pain was preceded by abdominal cramps and tenderness; after it began, she experienced nausea and vomiting accompanied by shoulder pain.
The nurse assesses a rapid, thready pulse; decreased blood pressure; and cold, diaphoretic extremities. The physician tentatively diagnoses a ruptured ectopic pregnancy. To prepare for Barbara's medical treatment, the nurse should implement which measures?

9. During her first prenatal examination, Catherine Greer, a 36-year-old gravida 4, para 1021 client, tells the nurse that her blood type is Rh negative and her husband's is Rh positive. Based on this information, the nurse should investigate which related history factors?

Multiple choice

10. What is the leading cause of maternal death during the first trimester?
(a) septic abortion
(b) choriocarcinoma
(c) hemorrhage from incomplete abortion
(d) ectopic pregnancy

11. Which of the following conditions does *not* increase the risk of early pregnancy loss?
    (a) hyperemesis gravidarum
    (b) uterine defects
    (c) previous first-trimester loss
    (d) cigarette or alcohol abuse

12. Which of the following circumstances is *not* a contraindication for tocolytic therapy to prevent preterm delivery?
    (a) chorioamnionitis
    (b) severe PIH
    (c) cervical dilation of less than 5 cm
    (d) fetal distress

Study questions

13. Briefly define PROM, and describe the maternal, fetal, and neonatal risks associated with it.

14. Which disorders can mimic a ruptured ectopic pregnancy, possibly complicating the diagnosis?

15. Identify at least four causes of recurrent (habitual) abortion.

16. Briefly describe the McDonald procedure used to correct an incompetent cervix. How early in a pregnancy can this procedure be performed?

17. What are the potential consequences of untreated hyperemesis gravidarum? When this condition is suspected, the nurse should assess for which signs and symptoms?

18. List at least six medical, obstetric, or social factors that may contribute to the onset of preterm labor and delivery.

19. Describe the adverse effects of beta-adrenergic agonists, used to treat preterm labor.

20. Early detection of PIH is a major goal of prenatal care. Briefly describe the use of mean arterial pressure (MAP) in determining PIH, as reported by Remich and Youngkin. Discuss some nursing implications of monitoring MAP changes during pregnancy.

21. Identify three factors that have significantly reduced the mortality rate for hemolytic disease of the newborn.

True or false

22. More than 75% of spontaneous abortions occur before 12 weeks' gestation.
    ❑ True ❑ False

23. Women with a history of ectopic pregnancy are not at increased risk for another.
    ❑ True ❑ False

24. Although preterm delivery is relatively rare, it accounts for most neonatal deaths.
❏ True ❏ False

25. With an incompetent cervix, dilation progresses painlessly and no uterine contractions occur.
❏ True ❏ False

26. Hypertension is the leading cause of maternal mortality in the United States.
❏ True ❏ False

27. Researchers have determined that hyperemesis gravidarum is a psychosomatic phenomenon.
❏ True ❏ False

28. A positive culdocentesis (aspiration of nonclotting blood) indicates an ectopic pregnancy.
❏ True ❏ False

◆ CHAPTER 24 ◆

PHYSIOLOGY OF LABOR AND CHILDBIRTH

CHAPTER OVERVIEW

Labor and childbirth result from an interplay of anatomic and physiologic changes within the mother and the fetus. To provide optimal care to the intrapartal client, the nurse must possess a thorough understanding of this interplay. Chapter 24 offers the necessary knowledge base. It discusses theories of labor initiation, then describes premonitory signs and symptoms of labor. It explores the mechanism of labor, correlating it with cervical changes, and details the cardinal movements of the fetus. After describing the events that occur during each stage of labor, the chapter investigates factors affecting labor, such as the fetus, the pelvis, and maternal psychological response. Finally, it summarizes maternal and fetal systemic responses to labor.

STUDENT ACTIVITIES

To test your familiarity with the information in this chapter, complete the following activities.

Clinical simulations

1. During a childbirth education class, Melinda Erickson, the nurse-educator, asks class members who have experienced labor to describe the body changes that preceded it. List at least five premonitory signs and symptoms that these class members would identify.

2. In Melinda's childbirth education class, Bill describes the false alarms that preceded the birth of his son 2 years earlier. He reports that he took his wife Cindy to the health care facility twice before she finally went into labor. Cindy, a gravida 3, para 1011 client, adds that she had increasing contractions every 10 to 20 minutes over a period of several hours. How should Melinda explain these contractions and describe their function in preparing the body for true labor?

3. After examining Sharon, a primigravid client age 19, to determine her labor status, the physician informs her that she is 5 cm dilated and 100% effaced. Because she never has attended a childbirth preparation class, Sharon does not understand these terms. How should the nurse explain their meaning?

4. During a prenatal visit to the nurse-midwife at 34 weeks' gestation, Debra and her husband Stephen ask many questions about how the neonate will move through her pelvis during labor and child-

birth. What factors should the nurse-midwife mention that help increase the pelvic diameters and promote labor and childbirth?

5. When enlisting Brad's aid in timing his partner Lisa's contractions during early labor, the nurse asks him to record the frequency and duration of Lisa's contractions. How should the nurse explain these terms to him?

6. Penny, a primigravid client age 18, telephones the labor room nurse; she states that she thinks she is in early labor, then asks how to proceed. After the nurse provides instructions, Penny asks if she can eat dinner before leaving for the health care facility. The nurse advises her not to eat, but encourages her to sip fluids. Why?

Multiple choice

7. Which of the following statements does *not* describe lightening, the subjective sensation that occurs late in pregnancy? Explain your answer.
(a) The client has a great burst of energy and may feel compelled to clean house to prepare for the neonate's arrival.
(b) About 2 weeks before going into labor, the client feels as though the fetus has "dropped."
(c) The client feels as if she can breathe easier and eat more at each meal
(d) The client feels a more frequent urge to urinate because of increased pelvic pressure.

8. Of the following statements, which one accurately describes spontaneous rupture of the membranes (SROM)?
(a) SROM is easy to recognize because nothing can mimic it.
(b) Most women have SROM before they go into labor.
(c) The client should wait until SROM occurs before going to the health care facility because it is the only sure sign of true labor.
(d) If a client does not give birth within 24 hours after SROM, she and her neonate are at increased risk for infection.

9. Cardinal movements refer to:
(a) the progressive stages of labor
(b) typical maternal positional changes during labor
(c) changes in cervical movement in response to fetal axis pressure
(d) the typical sequence of fetal positional changes during labor and childbirth.

10. Which of the following is *not* a part of the bony pelvis? Explain your answer.
(a) sacrum
(b) coccyx
(c) trochanter
(d) innominate bones

Study questions

11. Describe the nitrazine, ferning, and pooling tests used to determine whether SROM has occurred.

12. Arrange the following cardinal movements in the proper correct chronological order: internal rotation, descent, extension, flexion, expulsion, and external rotation.

13. Which forces result in fetal descent?

14. Briefly describe two functions of the sutures of the fetal skull during childbirth.

15. Describe the vertex attitude of the fetus.

16. List at least five predisposing factors in a fetal shoulder presentation (transverse lie).

17. Identify the three planes of the true pelvis, and explain their significance during labor and childbirth.

18. Which pelvic landmarks palpated during a vaginal examination indicate that the fetus is at O station? Why is palpation of these pelvic landmarks significant?

19. What are the three phases of a uterine contraction?

20. Identify three conditions that cause placental malfunction, thereby compromising fetal well-being.

21. Why should the nurse wait until a contraction is completed before taking the blood pressure of a client in labor?

22. Explain why the nurse should encourage the client to empty her bladder every 2 hours during labor.

Fill in the blank

23. Descent refers to ____________ of the fetus into the pelvic passageway.

24. When the fetal presenting part moves freely above the pelvic inlet before descent, it is said to be ____________ .

25. The fetus's head is delivered by the mechanism of ____________ in response to pressure from uterine contractions, resistance from the pelvic floor, and intra-abdominal pressure.

26. When the fetus's head passes over the perineum, rotates 45 degrees, and returns to the position it originally assumed during engagement, ____________ has occurred.

27. External rotation positions the fetus's shoulders in line with the ____________ diameter of the client's pelvis.

28. Once the shoulders pass the maternal perineum, the remainder of the body is delivered by the mechanism of ___________.

29. The period that begins immediately after birth and ends with expulsion of the placenta is called the ___________ stage of labor.

30. During the first stage of labor, the fetal scalp capillary blood pH is approximately ___________; during the second stage, it is approximately ___________.

31. A fetal scalp capillary blood pH value below ___________ indicates fetal distress.

Matching terms and definitions

32. Match each definition in the left column with the corresponding term in the right column.

(1) relationship of the parts of the fetus to one another	(a) attitude
(2) relationship of the landmark on the fetal presenting part to the front, back, and sides of the maternal pelvis	(b) biparietal diameter
(3) portion of the fetus that first enters the pelvic passageway	(c) breech presentation
(4) greatest transverse distance between the two parietal bones	(d) fetal lie
(5) relationship of the presenting part to the ischial spines	(e) fetal position
(6) fetal position in which the buttocks or the feet present first	(f) fontanel
(7) nonossified area of connective tissue between the skull bones where the sutures intersect	(g) presenting part
(8) relationship of the long axis of the fetus to the long axis of the mother	(h) station

Labeling illustrations

33. On this illustration of the fetal skull, indicate the three sets of bones, two fontanels, and four sutures.

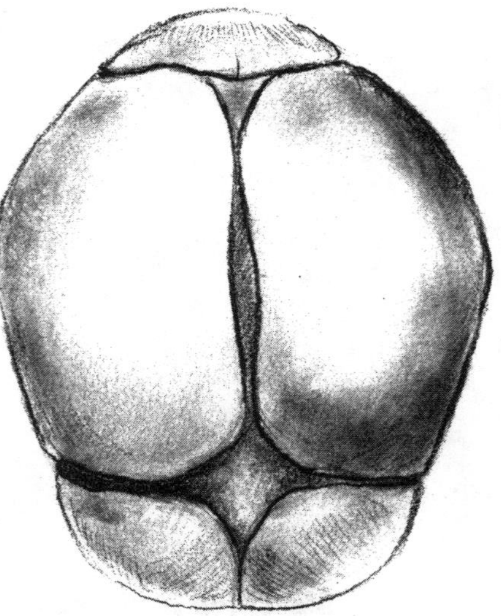

34. Label the illustrations below with the correct fetal presentation or position. Where appropriate, provide the proper abbreviation.

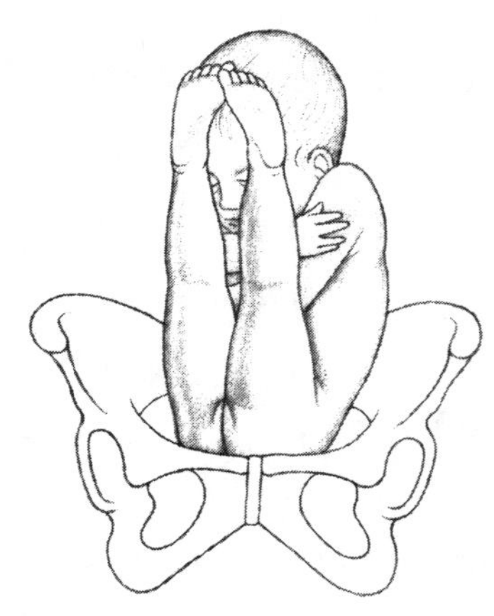

Illustration **A**__________

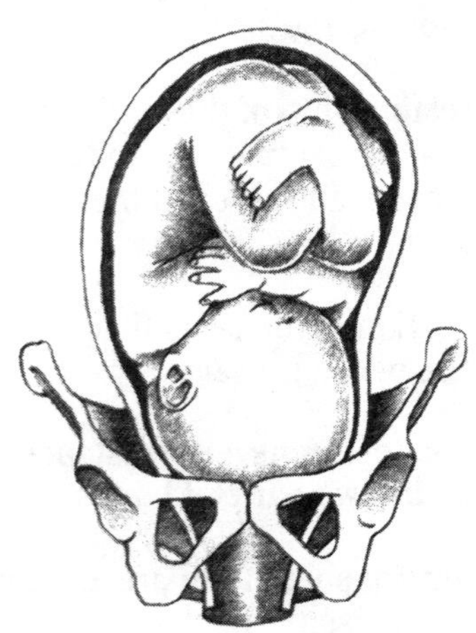

Illustration **B**__________

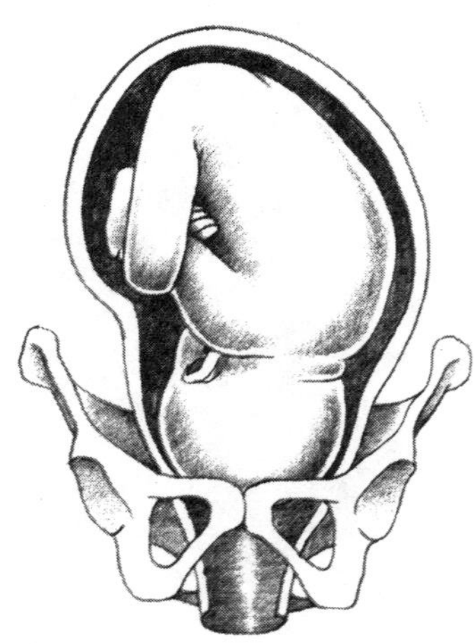

Illustration **C**__________

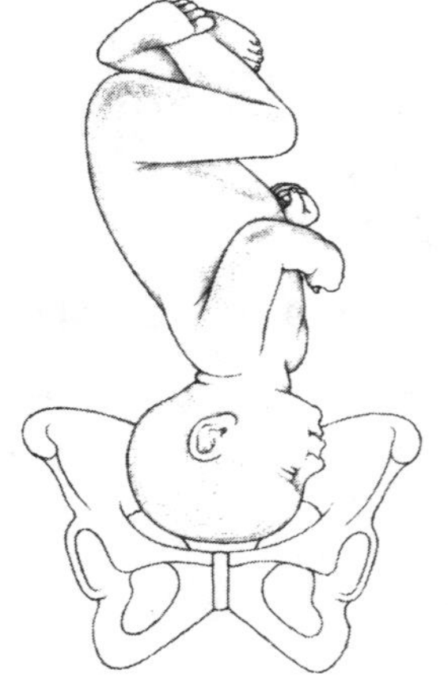

Illustration **D**__________

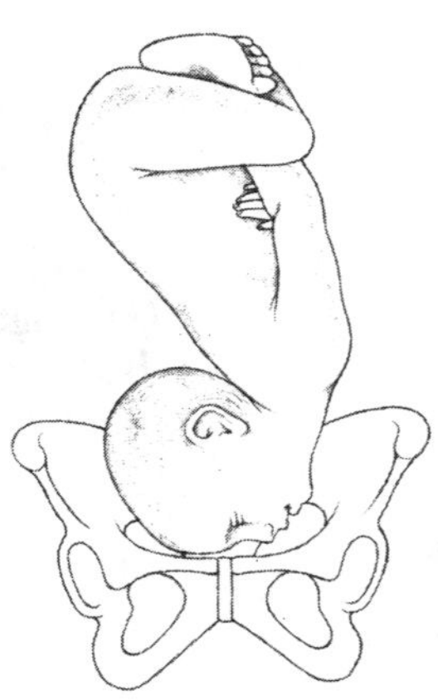

Illustration **E**__________

◆ CHAPTER 25 ◆

FETAL ASSESSMENT

CHAPTER OVERVIEW

To evaluate fetal well-being and detect fetal compromise promptly during the intrapartal period, the nurse must be familiar with the complex concepts and techniques central to fetal assessment. Chapter 25 provides basic guidelines for accurate interpretation of fetal heart rate patterns. It starts by exploring the relationship between uteroplacental-fetal circulation and fetal heart rate (FHR) regulation—the physiologic basis of fetal monitoring. Then it describes fetal and uterine monitoring techniques, examining the use of the fetoscope and the ultrasound stethoscope, discussing external and internal electronic fetal monitoring, and touching on related controversies. The chapter discusses FHR patterns, explaining how to recognize fetal distress patterns, and reviews fetal scalp blood sampling and other fetal assessment techniques. Finally, it outlines nursing responsibilities related to fetal assessment, including client teaching and support, accurate documentation, and legal responsibilities.

STUDENT ACTIVITIES

To test your familiarity with the information in this chapter, complete the following activities.

Clinical simulations

1. A primigravid client age 38, Jayne Wagner is admitted to the labor and delivery area in active labor. She complains of marked discomfort and requests epidural anesthesia. Initial evaluation of the FHR via internal fetal monitoring reveals baseline bradycardia with poor beat-to-beat long-term and short-term variability. Because of these findings, Jayne's physician decides against epidural anesthesia. What is the rationale for this decision?

2. Marianne, age 27, is a gravida 2, para 1001 client at 40 weeks' gestation admitted for induction of labor with oxytocin. Throughout her second and third trimesters, she has been monitored for gestational diabetes; for the past week, she has been followed closely for a slight rise in blood pressure. Several hours after admission, pelvic examination reveals that Marianne's cervix is dilated 3 cm. After performing an amniotomy, which reveals meconium-stained amniotic fluid, the physician applies an internal fetal scalp monitor. Three hours later, the nurse notes uterine hyperstimulation on the monitor strip accompanied by subtle, persistent, late decelerations. Explain the clinical significance of these decelerations, and state which actions, if any, the nurse should take at this time.

Multiple choice

3. The most common cause of fetal tachycardia is:
   (a) uteroplacental compromise
   (b) internal fetal monitoring
   (c) a low uterine resting tone
   (d) maternal fever

4. FHR is regulated by all of the following *except:*
   (a) the autonomic nervous system
   (b) the reticular activating system
   (c) the sympathetic and parasympathetic nervous systems
   (d) chemoreceptors and baroreceptors

Study questions

5. Identify at least five factors that can affect uteroplacental-fetal circulation during labor.

6. Explain how the autonomic nervous system, chemoreceptors, and baroreceptors help regulate the FHR during labor.

7. How does a supine maternal position during labor affect fetal circulation?

8. Describe three devices that the nurse may use to assess FHR.

9. Why must the nurse monitor the uterine contraction pattern of a client in labor?

10. Which three methods can the nurse use to assess the uterine contraction pattern? Which method is most accurate?

11. List at least three signs of fetal hypoxia that may appear on a fetal monitor strip.

12. What are the two causes of decreased FHR variability that typically have a gradual onset and may pose a serious threat to the fetus? Which fetal compensatory mechanisms are involved?

13. Name three characteristics of a variable deceleration FHR pattern.

14. How does the fetal scalp stimulation test help assess fetal health?

15. List three general categories of items that the nurse must document on the fetal monitor strip as well as on the chart of the client in labor. Identify specific items to document.

Fill in the blank

16. The starting point for all fetal assessment is the ____________.

17. The proper time for establishing the baseline FHR is between uterine contractions, when no fetal ____________ is occurring.

True or false

18. Baseline bradycardia accompanied by late decelerations and flat variability is an ominous sign of advanced fetal distress.
   ❑ True ❑ False

19. When hypoxemia occurs, the fetus responds initially by increasing short-term and long-term FHR variability.
❑ True ❑ False

20. Assessment of fetal distress may be based solely on a marked decrease in FHR variability.
❑ True ❑ False

21. Early decelerations are affected by maternal oxygen administration or position changes.
❑ True ❑ False

22. Late decelerations are nonreassuring because they indicate uteroplacental insufficiency and inadequate oxygen exchange.
❑ True ❑ False

23. Variable decelerations are subtle periodic changes that occur after the peak of a contraction and recover slowly after the contraction is completed.
❑ True ❑ False

Matching terms and definitions

24. Match each glossary term in the left column with the corresponding definition in the right column.

(1) acceleration	(a) nonreassuring waveform of the FHR indicating placental insufficiency
(2) baseline fetal tachycardia	(b) innocuous waveform deceleration of the FHR that mirrors uterine contractions and typically occurs when the cervix is dilated 4 to 7 cm
(3) baseline fetal heart rate	(c) resting pulse of the fetus assessed between contractions and without fetal movement
(4) early deceleration	(d) beat-to-beat changes in the FHR that reflect the degree of balance between the sympathetic and parasympathetic nervous systems
(5) fetal scalp blood sampling	(e) decrease in the FHR from the baseline lasting several minutes or longer; occurs in response to sudden stimulation of the vagal system, such as uterine tachysystole, anesthetics, or maternal hypotension
(6) late deceleration	(f) baseline FHR exceeding 160 beats/minute

(7) prolonged deceleration	(g) test that uses a fetal scalp blood sample to evaluate the fetus's acid-base status during labor
(8) variability	(h) increase in the FHR from the baseline that lasts less than 15 minutes
(9) variable deceleration	(i) nonuniform deceleration pattern indicating cord compression of variable significance; the most common deceleration pattern in labor

◆ CHAPTER 26 ◆

COMFORT PROMOTION DURING LABOR AND CHILDBIRTH

CHAPTER OVERVIEW

Typically, the pregnant client anticipates labor pain with concern—and even anxiety. Although such pain takes a predictable course, each client perceives it differently. During labor and childbirth, the nurse conducts ongoing assessment of the client's comfort level, implements pain-control measures, and evaluates the effectiveness of these measures. To prepare the nurse to fulfill these roles, Chapter 26 explores the characteristics and causes of labor pain and explores the physical and psychosocial factors that affect pain perception. Then it presents nursing care to promote comfort. It describes how to determine a client's comfort-promotion needs by monitoring her response to pain; discusses comfort measures that reduce anxiety, promote hygiene, and aid relaxation; and explains how to provide nursing care for the unprepared client. The chapter examines the role of both nonpharmacologic and pharmacologic pain-control strategies.

STUDENT ACTIVITIES

To test your familiarity with the information in this chapter, complete the following activities.

Clinical simulations

1. Linda McPherson, a 38-year-old primigravid client at 40 weeks' gestation, arrives in the labor and delivery area with contractions every 5 minutes. She seems agitated, markedly anxious, and unable to cope with the pain. She and her husband Dan, who remains at her side, express concern that they did not attend childbirth preparation classes. Physical examination shows that Linda's cervix is dilated only 3 cm as she begins the active phase of labor. Why should the nurse be concerned about Linda's excessive anxiety? Which interventions can the nurse implement to reduce her anxiety?

2. Carol Sylvan arrives at the health care facility in early labor, talking cheerfully about the impending birth with her support person, Glenda. Carol copes well with contractions, performing the breathing exercises she learned in her childbirth preparation course. However, after several hours, her contractions become stronger and more frequent, and she begins to withdraw. She has trouble following instructions, grows irritable, and refuses to be touched. How should the nurse interpret Carol's behavior?

3. Cindy has attended childbirth preparation classes and had two previous uneventful labor experiences. Now, however, as she pro-

gresses through the active phase of labor, she experiences severe sacral pain (back labor) and tells the nurse that she cannot cope with the pain. What is the probable cause of Cindy's pain? What are some steps the nurse can take to help increase Cindy's comfort?

4. Within 5 minutes after receiving epidural anesthesia during active labor, Denise Taylor's blood pressure drops dramatically, and internal fetal monitoring shows decreased beat-to-beat variability with bradycardia. What condition is Denise experiencing, and which nursing interventions are warranted?

Multiple choice

5. The gate control theory of pain transmission supports many of the pain-management techniques used in childbirth preparation. Which of the following factors is *not* related to this theory? Explain your answer.
   (a) controlled breathing
   (b) endorphin release
   (c) distraction
   (d) tactile stimulation

6. Of the following, which is an expected fetal response to a narcotic agonist (such as meperidine) during labor?
   (a) decreased beat-to-beat heart rate variability
   (b) fetal tachycardia
   (c) increased accelerations with fetal movement
   (d) subtle late decelerations during contractions

7. Of the following, which is *not* an advantage of the I.V. route for administering analgesia to a client in labor? Explain your answer.
   (a) rapid onset of action
   (b) predictable action
   (c) smaller dosage needed
   (d) shorter administration time

Study questions

8. What techniques are used to promote relaxation during labor?

9. For each stage of labor, identify the primary causes and typical location of pain.

10. List at least five factors that can affect a client's perception of and ability to cope with labor pain.

11. Identify at least three medical procedures or actions that can increase client discomfort during labor.

12. Before administering pain-relief agents to a client in labor, the nurse must assess which key fetal factors? Provide rationales for your answer.

13. Describe how hygiene promotion increases client comfort during labor, and state at least three nursing interventions that promote hygiene.

14. Compare and contrast analgesia and anesthesia used to relieve labor pain.

15. In a childbirth education course, the nurse educator typically discusses pharmacologic pain-control options so that expectant couples can make informed decisions about such options before labor begins. When reviewing the benefits and risks of pharmacologic pain-control methods, the nurse educator should provide what information?

16. What are some regional anesthesia techniques commonly used during vaginal delivery?

17. Describe the epidural block, and discuss its advantages, disadvantages, and adverse effects.

18. When caring for a client experiencing labor pain, the nurse should document which items? (Assume the client received I.V. analgesia.)

Fill in the blank

19. The goal of relaxation techniques taught during childbirth preparation courses is to reduce ____________ and ____________, thereby helping to calm the mind and body.

20. Typically, relaxation techniques are effective because they distract the client from ____________, increase her sense of control over pain, and aid sleep and rest.

◆ CHAPTER 27 ◆

THE FIRST STAGE OF LABOR

CHAPTER OVERVIEW

Nursing care for the client, fetus, and family during the first stage of labor must address psychosocial and cultural concerns as well as physical needs. Chapter 27 details the required care, describing intrapartal nursing responsibilities before the client's admission to the labor and delivery area and continuing throughout the first stage of labor. It explains how to collect health history and physical assessment data to evaluate maternal and fetal status and to distinguish true labor from false labor. Then it discusses the additional data to collect after the client's admission—to incorporate further history, physical findings, and laboratory data and to integrate psychosocial and cultural needs into the client's care. After describing how to formulate nursing diagnoses, the chapter delineates the planning and implementation of initial and ongoing nursing care for the client in the first stage of labor. It explains how to recognize variations in this stage and provides appropriate interventions for such variations. It emphasizes nursing actions that ensure the safety of the mother and fetus, discusses comfort measures appropriate for the first stage, and explains how to ensure the client's and family's active participation during this time.

STUDENT ACTIVITIES

To test your familiarity with the information in this chapter, complete the following activities.

Clinical simulations

1. After 2 hours of observation, the nurse reevaluates Rona Byrd in the preadmission area of the labor and delivery unit to determine her labor status. A 23-year-old client at 38 weeks' gestation, Ms. Byrd has stable vital signs; fetal heart tones indicate a healthy fetus. Contractions are irregular, occurring every 4 to 12 minutes for a duration of 20 to 30 seconds, and are mild to palpation. Ms. Byrd reports abdominal pressure that decreases somewhat when she walks. Her membranes are intact, and no evidence of bloody show exists. Vaginal examination results remain unchanged, revealing cervical dilation of 1 cm, 25% effacement, and –2 station. Based on these assessment findings, should the nurse assume Ms. Byrd is in true labor? Explain your answer.

2. The nurse should give Ms. Byrd what instructions upon discharge?

3. Alicia Nordstrom, a new client, has just arrived at the labor and delivery area for admission. To help determine her labor status, the nurse collects her health history data. Prioritize Ms. Nordstrom's health history findings by placing a number from 1 to 12 by each

statement below, with *1* indicating the most important finding and *12* the least important.
(a) The fetus is active and moves every day.
(b) The client received prenatal care from nurse-midwives at the health department.
(c) Her contractions occur 4 to 5 minutes apart and last 45 to 60 seconds.
(d) Her labor began 5 hours ago.
(e) She is a primigravid client.
(f) She has been monitored closely for gestational diabetes and has achieved good blood glucose control through diet alone.
(g) Her mother has accompanied her to the health care facility.
(h) Her membranes ruptured 45 minutes ago; she reports a clear, pink-tinged fluid.
(i) She is 15 years old and single.
(j) She reports no vaginal bleeding.
(k) Based on her expected delivery date, she now is at 40 weeks' gestation.
(l) She is in good health with no significant medical history.

4. When reviewing Ms. Nordstrom's antepartal chart, the nurse notes the following laboratory data:
ABO blood type and Rh type: O positive
Antibody screening test (indirect Coombs' test): negative
Rubella antibodies test: immune
VDRL test or rapid plasma reagin (RPR) test: nonreactive
Papanicolaou (Pap) smear: Class I
Which studies are missing from this list of routinely ordered tests for a client in labor? Explain how these missing studies can help assess Ms. Nordstrom and her fetus.

5. To examine Ms. Nordstrom, the nurse performs Leopold's maneuvers. Explain the purpose of these maneuvers.

6. The nurse examining Ms. Nordstrom palpates the fetal head in the fundus and auscultates fetal heart tones above the umbilicus. Based on these findings, which fetal presentation exists?

7. Jeanette Green, a multigravid client, is entering transition (the final part of the active phase of the first stage of labor). The nurse should assess vital signs, contractions, and fetal heart tones how frequently?

8. Mary O'Brien has planned a family-centered, birthing-room labor and delivery with her husband, mother, and 6-year-old son present. List five interventions the nurse could implement to promote the effective involvement of Mary's husband during the first stage of labor and three interventions to promote the effective involvement of her mother and son.

Study questions

9. Identify the two major goals of nursing assessment for a new client admitted to the labor and delivery area.

10. Describe at least four ways in which the nurse can increase client comfort during and after a vaginal examination.

11. Which conditions can mimic true labor?

12. How is true labor distinguished from false labor?

13. When assessing a client who reports spontaneous rupture of the membranes, the nurse should question her about which factors?

14. Describe some nursing measures that promote comfort for a client in active labor, and explain why these measures are important.

15. When documenting vaginal examination findings, the nurse should include what information?

Fill in the blank

16. The first stage of labor begins with the onset of regular, rhythmic ____________ and ends with complete cervical ____________.

17. Lack of progressive cervical change commonly leads to determination of ____________.

True or false

18. In most clients with term pregnancies, premature rupture of the membranes precedes the onset of labor.
❑ True ❑ False

19. During active labor, the occiput posterior position of the fetus slows labor progress.
❑ True ❑ False

20. To determine rupture of the membranes, the nurse first performs a vaginal examination.
❑ True ❑ False

21. The examiner must use an electronic fetal monitor to diagnose fetal distress.
❑ True ❑ False

22. A fetal heart rate of 120 to 160 beats/minute indicates absence of fetal distress.
❑ True ❑ False

Matching terms and definitions

23. Match each definition in the left column with the corresponding term in the right column.

(1) relationship of the fetal long axis to the maternal long axis	(a) amniotomy
(2) blood-tinged vaginal discharge occurring at the onset of labor when the cervical mucus plug is dislodged and small cervical capillaries break	(b) effleurage

(3) light fingertip massage	(c) first stage of labor
(4) artificial rupture of amniotic membranes	(d) molding
(5) descent of the fetal presenting part into the maternal pelvis	(e) station
(6) relationship of the leading fetal presenting part to a point on the maternal pelvis	(f) ferning
(7) microscopic pattern found in a smear of dried amniotic fluid indicating rupture of the amniotic membranes	(g) bloody show
(8) relationship of the fetal presenting part to the ischial spines of the maternal pelvis	(h) effacement
(9) onset of regular, rhythmic uterine contractions leading to complete cervical dilation	(i) position
(10) shaping of the fetus's head by overlapping of the sutures, which helps the head conform to the birth canal	(j) caput succedaneum
	(k) engagement
	(l) presentation
	(m) lie

◆ CHAPTER 28 ◆

THE SECOND STAGE OF LABOR

CHAPTER OVERVIEW

Nursing care during the second stage of labor requires both active encouragement and continuous assessment of maternal expulsive efforts and fetal response. Chapter 28 discusses the characteristics of the second stage and examines the multiple factors that affect its progress. It describes the signs that mark onset of the second stage, compares and contrasts the two phases of this stage, and explores the factors influencing its duration. After discussing ongoing nursing assessment of a client and her fetus during bearing-down efforts, the chapter reviews nursing strategies used to enhance maternal efficiency. It explores nursing responsibilities during delivery, and provides specific care guidelines for the neonate immediately after delivery, including assignment of an Apgar score.

STUDENT ACTIVITIES

To test your familiarity with the information in this chapter, complete the following activities.

Clinical simulations

1. Latoya Madison, age 23, is a primigravid client who has been in active labor since her membranes ruptured spontaneously with clear fluid early this morning. On her admission, maternal and fetal vital signs are stable; pelvic examination reveals cervical dilation of 7 cm. One hour later, Ms. Madison begins to grunt involuntarily and bear down during contractions. Reexamination reveals that her cervix is dilated only 8 cm and that the fetus is in a posterior position, causing a premature urge to push. Explain why the nurse should try to discourage Ms. Madison from bearing down at this time, and describe some appropriate nursing actions.

2. Rose Ciliberto and her husband Bill attended childbirth preparation classes together and wish to participate in the birth of their second child as much as possible. After her admission to the labor and delivery unit this morning, Ms. Ciliberto passed through an uneventful first stage of labor. Now, during the second stage, she is encouraged to use open-glottis pushing. As delivery becomes imminent, she assumes a lateral recumbent position as she and Bill discussed previously with the nurse-midwife. List four advantages and four disadvantages of this nontraditional labor position.

3. Todd Williams is born by normal spontaneous vaginal delivery over an intact perineum. After positioning him under a radiant heat warmer, the nurse conducts an assessment, which reveals a heart rate of 120 beats/minute, a somewhat slow and irregular respiratory effort, some flexion of the extremities, grimacing after stimula-

tion with a bulb syringe, and acrocyanosis. Based on these findings, the nurse should assign which Apgar score and should take which actions, if any?

4. During a childbirth preparation course, Diane Albrecht, the nurse-educator, prepares expectant couples for the possibility of an episiotomy. Ms. Albrecht should mention which four potential benefits of this procedure?

Study questions

5. An experienced intrapartal nurse can recognize completion of the first stage of labor by observing for classic signs of the second stage. Identify at least five such signs.

6. Some authorities divide the second stage into two distinct phases. State when each phase ends and describe the sensations the client feels during each phase.

7. List at least five fetal factors and five maternal factors that may affect duration of the second stage.

8. What are some causes of the variations in FHR patterns commonly seen during the second stage?

9. Although authorities disagree on the effects of a prolonged second stage, some suggest a correlation between an unusually long second stage and certain poor maternal and neonatal outcomes. Identify some of these adverse outcomes.

10. To determine a neonate's Apgar score, the nurse immediately should assess which five factors?

Fill in the blank

11. The second stage of labor begins with complete ___________ and culminates in ___________ .

12. The nurse should suspect an abnormality if no fetal descent occurs after a primigravid client bears down for ___________ hour or after a multiparous client bears down for ___________ minutes.

13. A change in amniotic fluid color during the second stage may indicate ___________ .

14. Some authorities consider abnormal a second stage that lasts longer than __________ .

◆ CHAPTER 29 ◆

THE THIRD AND FOURTH STAGES OF LABOR

CHAPTER OVERVIEW

During the third and fourth stages of labor—a period extending from the neonate's delivery to approximately 1 hour after delivery of the placenta—the client and neonate experience crucial physiologic adaptations. Chapter 29 prepares the nurse to care for a client and her neonate during this time, detailing the separate management required for each. It stresses evaluation of maternal vital signs, placental status and delivery, and the perineum during the third stage. Then it describes nursing measures that promote hygiene, proper positioning, neonatal care, and parent-infant bonding. It briefly explains how to assess the neonate and how to palpate and massage the client's uterus after delivery. Then it outlines nursing care during the fourth stage. It explains how to assess the client for discomfort and recovery from anesthesia or analgesia as well as how to evaluate her response to childbirth and her neonate. Then the chapter discusses key interventions, such as preventing hemorrhage and maintaining maternal hygiene and comfort. It highlights family-centered care, emphasizing how the nurse promotes parent-infant bonding.

STUDENT ACTIVITIES

To test your familiarity with the information in this chapter, complete the following activities.

1. Kate Pavlick, a primigravid client age 24, has just completed a long, difficult labor marked by several episodes of transient fetal distress. Fortunately, these episodes resolved without the need for surgery. At delivery, meconium-stained amniotic fluid appeared; the neonate had a low birth weight. Discuss some findings that the nurse might identify when inspecting the placenta, and explain the significance of these findings.

2. Judy Bixler, a gravida 6, para 5005 client, is admitted to the labor and delivery area in active labor at 37 weeks' gestation. Her records indicate that she has gestational diabetes and was diagnosed with hydramnios and a large-for-gestational-age fetus 1 week before admission. Her previous neonates were large at birth, and Judy had heavy bleeding during her last delivery.
   After many hours, Judy's labor becomes arrested; the physician initiates oxytocin to augment labor. After an extended delay, Judy finally progresses to the second stage. However, she must deliver

with the aid of forceps, resulting in vaginal trauma. Identify at least five factors that place Judy at high risk for postpartal hemorrhage.

3. During the fourth stage of labor, the nurse palpates Sharon Mitford's uterus and finds that the fundus is boggy and located two fingerbreadths above the umbilicus, deviated to the right of midline. The nurse should suspect which conditions as possible causes of these findings and should carry out which measures?

4. One hour after her neonate was delivered, Laura Ritter complains of throbbing perineal pain. Examining her perineum, the nurse finds a large, purplish mass at the vaginal introitus. The nurse institutes comfort measures, but Laura remains agitated and restless. Her vital signs reveal tachycardia and decreasing blood pressure. The nurse should suspect which condition?

5. Mai and Poy Peng, recent arrivals from Thailand, are first-time parents. Just after Ms. Peng's uneventful labor and delivery, she and Mr. Peng gaze quietly at their newborn son while her episiotomy is being repaired. The nurse overhears Ms. Peng say, "He looks just like his father" and "What beautiful eyes he has." Ms. Peng holds her son so that she can touch his face and look directly at him. She reaches out with her fingertips, then begins to stroke him. Which process does Ms. Peng's behavior demonstrate? Identify the position in which she is holding her son, and discuss its significance.

Multiple choice

6. After completion of the third stage of labor, expected blood loss measures:
(a) greater than 500 ml
(b) less than 500 ml
(c) greater than 750 ml
(d) less than 200 ml

7. During the third stage, the nurse evaluates the client for all of the following *except:*
(a) homeostasis
(b) placental status and delivery
(c) cervical lacerations
(d) perineal repair

8. Which of the following is *not* an expected finding during inspection of the placenta? Explain your answer.
(a) smooth, rounded edges throughout
(b) a thick, lobulated maternal side
(c) battledore insertion of the cord
(d) two umbilical vessels

Study questions

9. How long does the third stage of labor typically last?

10. List the normal signs of placental separation.

11. Briefly describe the two mechanisms of placental expulsion.

12. What are the nurse's responsibilities when assisting with episiotomy repair?

13. Briefly describe the immediate physiologic changes associated with postpartal hemorrhage and identify the common causes of this complication.

14. Identify the three key components of neonatal nursing care immediately after delivery.

15. Explain why thermoregulation is essential to the neonate, and discuss some nursing measures to prevent hypothermia.

16. Describe appropriate nursing interventions during the fourth stage of labor.

17. How often should the nurse perform physical assessment on a client during the fourth stage of labor? What should this assessment include?

18. Define paternal engrossment, and describe typical engrossment behaviors.

19. What are the three common causes of an elevated maternal temperature during the fourth stage of labor?

◆ CHAPTER 30 ◆

FAMILY SUPPORT DURING THE INTRAPARTAL PERIOD

CHAPTER OVERVIEW

Support plays a key role in increasing client comfort and reducing emotional stress during labor and delivery. Chapter 30 discusses the principles of support during the intrapartal period and examines various ways in which support can be provided to both the client and her family. It explores the physical and emotional benefits of support and delineates the sources of support that may be available to a client, including her partner, parents, children, other family members, and friends. After reviewing cultural considerations relevant to client support, the chapter investigates the nurse's role in providing support, such as offering direct support and assisting the client's primary support person to function effectively. It reviews nursing measures that help the client's family and support person as well as interventions that help balance the client's needs against the needs of others during labor and delivery.

STUDENT ACTIVITIES

To test your familiarity with the information in this chapter, complete the following activities.

Clinical simulations

1. Lisa Mervis, age 18, is a primigravid client in early labor who seems fearful and anxious as she is admitted to the labor and delivery area. The nurse asks if a relative or friend has come with her. Lisa replies tearfully that only her mother has come because her boyfriend suddenly changed his mind about being with her during labor. Her mother states that she wants to stay with Lisa, even though she has not attended childbirth preparation classes. Assuming that Lisa wants her mother to stay, identify at least three benefits she may gain from her mother's ongoing support.

2. Stephanie Klein, a primigravid client age 34, is in active labor. As the nurse enters the room to assess her labor progress, Ms. Klein's partner, Justin, is reading a newspaper at the bedside, seemingly disinterested. Ms. Klein tells the nurse that she appreciates Justin's presence; she seems to be coping well and appears unconcerned that Justin is not involved more actively in her labor. Provide an explanation for Ms. Klein's satisfaction with Justin's level of support.

3. Although David Carr, an airline pilot, has not attended childbirth classes with his wife Betsy, he and Betsy express a strong desire to be together as she is admitted to the labor and delivery area in ac-

tive labor. Describe four ways in which David can serve as a valuable support person for Betsy during labor, despite his lack of training in relaxation techniques and breathing exercises.

4. Rosalind Graffeo, age 37, is a primigravid client who has chosen to give birth in a free-standing birth center so that she and her husband Steve can share the experience with their family and close friends. During labor, the visitors in Rosalind's room include Steve's and Rosalind's mothers and Steve's brother and his girlfriend, who are taking photographs. As Rosalind's labor becomes more active, she grows more introspective and less social and has trouble concentrating on her breathing techniques. The visitors, however, remain engrossed in the drama of the event and talk noisily in her room. Rosalind becomes increasing uncomfortable with the distractions, and her labor progress is impeded. The nurse should take which action at this time?

5. When orienting a new group of graduate nurses to the labor and delivery area, Patty Wilmer, the in-service educator, emphasizes the importance of showing sensitivity to all client needs—psychological as well as physical—when planning and implementing care. To improve the nurses' understanding of client needs for labor support, Ms. Wilmer presents the following list of supportive nursing behaviors during labor and asks the students to rank these behaviors from most helpful to least helpful (based on the 1987 study by Kintz). Indicate how the students should rank these behaviors by placing a number from 1 to 7 in front of each phrase below, with *1* indicating the most helpful behavior and *7* the least helpful.
(a) providing for the needs of the support person
(b) providing friendly and personal care
(c) familiarizing the client with her surroundings
(d) coaching
(e) accepting the client's behavior
(f) making the client feel cared about as an individual
(g) praising the client's efforts

Study questions

6. Define the concept of support.

7. Identify four common sources of support for the client in labor.

8. Why must the nurse tailor specific strategies for client and family support to the client's individual needs?

9. Briefly describe the benefits of using touch to show support to the client in labor, and state how the nurse can encourage a support person to show caring through the use of touch (assuming that the client is receptive to such support).

10. Because cultural preferences influence a client's choice of labor support person, nurses must be especially sensitive to the needs of clients whose cultural backgrounds differ from their own. Contrast

the typical support-person preferences of a Korean-American client with those of a Mexican-American client. (Also consider whether and how these preferences differ from your own.)

11. Define birth culture, and explain its role in the birth process.

12. The nurse should focus on what major issues when assessing the needs and concerns of a client's primary support person?

◆ CHAPTER 31 ◆

HIGH-RISK INTRAPARTAL CLIENTS

CHAPTER OVERVIEW

During labor and delivery, various conditions may jeopardize the health of the client, fetus, or neonate. Nursing care for the client with such a condition poses a challenge because it demands advanced clinical knowledge and skills as well as familiarity with the technology used to improve perinatal outcome. Chapter 31 explores selected high-risk intrapartal conditions—age-related concerns, cardiac disease, diabetes mellitus, infection, substance abuse, pregnancy-induced hypertension (PIH), and isoimmunization. It examines the stressors affecting the high-risk intrapartal client and describes the perinatal problems that may result from inadequate prenatal care. Then it outlines the responsibilities of the nurse caring for the high-risk intrapartal client. The chapter delineates the maternal, fetal, and neonatal risk factors associated with selected high-risk conditions. It explains how to adapt the nursing process and tailor normal intrapartal care to meet this client's special needs. It also discusses management of various intrapartal emergencies.

STUDENT ACTIVITIES

To test your familiarity with the information in this chapter, complete the following activities.

Clinical simulations

1. After 12 years of marriage, Courtney Duncan and her husband Jeff recently decided to have a child. Courtney, age 41, is a successful insurance broker in good health. She has had early and regular prenatal care to maintain a healthy first pregnancy. An amniocentesis, which revealed that the fetus was a girl, was normal.
   The Duncans are well prepared for childbirth. After attending a series of childbirth classes, they formulated a plan whose goals included a natural labor experience without unnecessary use of invasive procedures or medications.
   At 39 weeks' gestation, Courtney is admitted to the labor and delivery unit with regular, moderately intense contractions occurring 3 to 4 minutes apart and lasting for 1 minute. Examination reveals complete cervical effacement with 5 cm dilation and a minus 2 station. The fetus is in a cephalic presentation and an occiput posterior position. Courtney reports that her labor pain is mostly in her back. Jeff remains supportive and concerned. Based on these admission assessment findings, briefly identify Courtney's intrapartal nursing needs.

2. After several hours, Courtney's contractions become much less efficient, her cervix shows lack of progressive dilation, and fetal descent is absent. Thus, despite their initial birth goals, she and Jeff

consent when the physician recommends oxytocin augmentation related to a diagnosis of secondary arrest of labor.
Identify the factors that contributed to Courtney's arrested labor, and explain why labor dysfunction is relatively common in mature clients such as Courtney.

3. Once Courtney's labor dysfunction pattern is identified, the nurse should expect to implement which measures?

4. Courtney finally progresses to the second stage of labor after a long, exhausting first stage. She has been pushing for 2½ hours when the physician suggests a vacuum extraction to assist delivery. Explain why this procedure is more common in mature clients, and name the related complication the nurse should assess Courtney for after delivery.

5. Trudi Simone, a multigravid client age 26 with insulin-dependent diabetes, is admitted to the labor and delivery area in active labor. During the nursing admission assessment, she reports that she had persistent nausea and vomiting all night and states that she did not take her morning dose of insulin. She seems somewhat confused and slightly breathless; her breath has a fruity odor. The nurse measures a blood pressure of 90/50 mm Hg and notes that her skin is dry and flushed. The nurse should suspect which condition as the cause of these assessment findings? Explain why this suspected condition constitutes an obstetric emergency.

6. To ensure the safety of Ms. Simone and her fetus, the nurse should take what steps?

7. Henrietta Caruthers, age 23, is admitted to the labor and delivery area in active labor. She complains of a severe headache and blurry vision; she states that she has not received prenatal care.
The nurse measures the following vital signs: blood pressure of 160/110 mm Hg, a pulse rate of 88 beats/minute, a respiratory rate of 24 breaths/minute, and a temperature of 99.2° F. Mrs. Caruthers's contractions are strong, occurring 2 minutes apart. Her fundal height measures only 32 cm, although she is at 40 weeks' gestation by the date of her last menstrual period (LMP). The fetus weighs an estimated 5 lb. The nurse also assesses marked edema and brisk reflexes, with three-beat ankle clonus. A catheterized urine specimen shows 2+ proteinuria. Which condition do Mrs. Caruthers's history and physical findings suggest? The nurse should anticipate what potential complications of this condition for Mrs. Caruthers and her fetus or neonate?

8. Mrs. Caruther's physician diagnoses severe preeclampsia. Which four goals should guide her nursing care?

9. On admission to the labor and delivery area, Candy Burnes, a single primigravid client age 15, complains of abdominal cramps and influenza-like symptoms, including chills and fever. Thirty-five weeks pregnant by the date of her LMP, she tells the nurse that "water" has been leaking from her vagina for the past few days; she ex-

plains that she did not seek evaluation for this problem because she "wasn't having labor pains yet."

Physical assessment reveals a temperature of 100.2° F, a pulse rate of 102 beats/minute, a respiratory rate of 24 breaths/minute, and blood pressure of 100/60 mm Hg. Abdominal examination shows a single fetus weighing an estimated 4½ to 5 lb. Candy's abdomen is slightly warm and tender to the touch on palpation. The external monitor shows mild contractions every 2 to 3 minutes, each lasting 30 to 40 seconds; the fetal heart rate ranges from 170 to 180 beats/minute. Speculum examination reveals ruptured membranes; the fluid has a slightly foul odor.

The physician makes a presumptive diagnosis of intrapartal infection. Identify the risk factors for intrapartal infection in Candy's history and physical findings.

10. Candy's physician confirms infection—specifically, chorioamnionitis, an inflammation of the fetal membranes. Briefly discuss the nursing care Candy will require.

Study questions

11. Briefly describe the physiologic implications of labor for a pregnant client with cardiac disease.

12. Why should the nurse discourage a client with cardiac disease from bearing down during the second stage of labor?

13. Explain why the nurse should anticipate psychosocial problems for the healthy adolescent during labor and delivery, even if she had no antepartal complications.

14. When evidence of substance abuse exists, the nurse must stay alert for which major intrapartal risks?

15. Briefly describe the signs and symptoms of PIH, and identify their physiologic bases.

16. How is the diagnosis of PIH confirmed?

17. What is the treatment of choice for seizure prevention in a client with preeclampsia? How does this treatment achieve the desired effect?

18. What are the signs of magnesium sulfate toxicity? What preparation is prescribed for a magnesium sulfate overdose?

19. Explain why the nurse must address the needs of the family of the high-risk intrapartal client.

◆ CHAPTER 32 ◆

SPECIAL OBSTETRIC PROCEDURES

CHAPTER OVERVIEW

To help ensure a positive delivery outcome, some clients require special obstetric interventions, ranging from relatively conventional procedures (such as labor induction, amniotomy, and episiotomy) to cesarean delivery and other higher-risk techniques. These procedures have led to increased obstetric nursing responsibilities: Besides understanding their indications, contraindications, and risks, the nurse must both possess the clinical skills to assist the obstetric team and the teaching skills to provide education to the client and her family. Chapter 32 discusses special obstetric procedures, then outlines related nursing care. It reviews the components of initial assessment, delineating the key baseline physical data to gather. Then it describes ongoing assessment during and after labor, pointing out how to adapt the assessment to the specific procedure performed. The chapter highlights nursing measures to maintain fluid balance, promote uterine contractions, prevent infection, and provide psychological support.

STUDENT ACTIVITIES

To test your familiarity with the information in this chapter, complete the following activities.

Clinical simulations

1. After years of infertility and eventual successful treatment with clomiphene citrate, Roberta Nabors is pregnant with twins. As her due date approaches, the physician determines that one fetus is in a stable vertex presentation but the other is in an unstable oblique lie. Consequently, she recommends cesarean delivery. Identify the risks of cesarean delivery that Roberta and her husband Steve must consider.

2. Hoping to avoid cesarean delivery because of its risks, Roberta and Steve ask the physician about the alternatives to surgical delivery. She tells them that without surgery, the second fetus may descend spontaneously into a vertex presentation after the first is delivered; however, it is just as likely that this fetus would require an emergency procedure called internal podalic version. How would the physician describe this procedure and its associated risks and complications?

3. After considering their options, Roberta and Steve consent to a cesarean delivery with regional anesthesia. On Roberta's admission to the labor and delivery area, the nurse determines that Roberta has

a nursing diagnosis of *fear related to the real or potential threat to her fetuses or herself.* How can the nurse help alleviate Roberta's fears and provide psychological support for her and Steve?

4. As Roberta is being prepared for surgery, she asks the nurse if she will be able to deliver vaginally after this cesarean delivery. How should the nurse respond?

5. Which criteria must be met for Roberta to have a vaginal birth after cesarean (VBAC) delivery during a subsequent pregnancy?

6. Twelve hours into labor, Candace Romero is making slow progress. During the second stage, 1 hour after she begins pushing, the physician decides to facilitate delivery with a vacuum extraction. How should the nurse explain this procedure to Mrs. Romero and her family?

7. Greta and Frank Bach are looking forward to the birth of their third child and only boy (identified on ultrasound). During a routine prenatal visit at 40 weeks' gestation, pelvic examination reveals that Greta is dilated 4 to 5 cm and that the fetus is in an engaged vertex presentation; however, she is not having contractions. After conferring, the nurse-midwife and physician suggest induction by amniotomy to promote a more predictable labor and delivery course. Before obtaining their consent, the nurse-midwife should discuss what major risks of this procedure with the Bachs?

8. A prenatal examination at 36 weeks' gestation reveals that the fetus of Alison Marks, a multigravid client, is in a breech presentation. To promote spontaneous version at home before her next office visit, the nurse might suggest which measures to Ms. Marks?

9. As Regina Donaldson progresses through the second stage of labor, her preterm fetus shows signs of acute distress. Determining that a rapid assisted vaginal delivery is necessary, the physician makes a mediolateral episiotomy and delivers the fetus using Tucker-McLean forceps. Explain the rationale for this approach.

Multiple choice

10. Immediately after an amniotomy, the nurse should:
    (a) assess maternal temperature and blood pressure
    (b) assess the frequency and intensity of uterine contractions
    (c) assess the fetal heart rate and amniotic fluid characteristics
    (d) assess maternal comfort level and coping skills.

11. Which of the following measures may help prevent vaginal lacerations or the need for an episiotomy during delivery?
    (a) diagonal curl exercise
    (b) pelvic tilt
    (c) Tailor squat exercise
    (d) perineal massage

12. During an assisted vaginal delivery, the nurse should anticipate the physician's need for Piper forceps in which of the following circumstances?

(a) to rotate a fetus from a persistent occiput posterior presentation to a position that better accommodates vaginal delivery
(b) to permit traction and flexion of the fetus's head during a breech delivery
(c) to facilitate a mid forceps rotation and delivery of a fetus in an occiput transverse position
(d) to allow for an episiotomy and a low-outlet, forceps delivery

Study questions

13. Which disadvantages are associated with the transverse lower uterine segment incision, recommended for a cesarean delivery?

14. Identify the indications for external version, and list the four conditions that help minimize complications of this procedure.

15. What are the two major medical considerations in labor induction?

16. Why must the nurse avoid administering large amounts of I.V. fluid to a client undergoing oxytocin labor induction?

17. List the benefits of an amniotomy.

18. What are the nurse's responsibilities during and after a forceps delivery?

True or false

19. External version is accomplished more easily in primiparous than multiparous clients.
❏ True ❏ False

20. Oxytocin infusion may cause excessive or tetanic uterine contractions.
❏ True ❏ False

21. Approximately 25% of low transverse cesarean incisions rupture during a subsequent vaginal delivery.
❏ True ❏ False

22. The classical incision used for a surgical delivery reduces the risk of rupture during subsequent pregnancy.
❏ True ❏ False

23. Dyspareunia indicates the need for an episiotomy.
❏ True ❏ False

24. Cesarean delivery is safer than mid or high forceps delivery.
❏ True ❏ False

◆ CHAPTER 33 ◆

INTRAPARTAL COMPLICATIONS

CHAPTER OVERVIEW

Chapter 33 discusses major intrapartal complications that can threaten the health and well-being of the client, her fetus, or both. It reviews the pathophysiology of complications stemming from reproductive system disorders and identifies the uterine, pelvic, placental, membrane and amniotic fluid, and umbilical cord factors that can cause intrapartal complications. Then it describes complications that involve the fetus directly. The chapter delineates the vital role of the nurse in detecting intrapartal complications, assisting in their resolution, and providing the client with appropriate physical and emotional care. It explains how to recognize complications promptly, prioritize needs when a complication becomes life-threatening, and apply the nursing process to promote an optimal outcome.

STUDENT ACTIVITIES

To test your familiarity with the information in this chapter, complete the following activities.

Clinical simulations

1. At 2 p.m., Igdalis Nacione is admitted to the labor and delivery area. Her contractions are occurring every 3 to 4 minutes, last 50 to 60 seconds, and are moderately intense. Pelvic examination reveals cervical dilation of 5 cm, 80% effacement, 0 station, and active labor. At 5 p.m., the contraction pattern becomes less frequent and intense; pelvic reexamination shows no change since the previous assessment. Ms. Nacione is experiencing which dysfunctional labor pattern? During which phase of the first stage of labor does this pattern typically occur?

2. Beth Drake, age 38, is admitted to the labor and delivery area at 35 weeks' gestation complaining of constant, severe abdominal pain. Her abdomen is rigid and boardlike; fetal assessment reveals severe fetal distress with pronounced tachycardia. Ms. Drake's vital signs indicate that she is developing shock. What is the most likely diagnosis of her condition?

3. Leslie Paulson, age 32, is 37 weeks pregnant with her fourth child when she arrives at the labor and delivery area. She expresses anxiety because she has felt no fetal movements for over 24 hours and now has what seem to be early labor pains. Initial nursing assessment reveals lack of fetal heart tones; ultrasound examination shows that the fetus is dead. Once Ms. Paulson and her family have been informed of the fetus's status, the nurse should take which actions?

Multiple choice

4. Which of the following factors does *not* cause dysfunctional labor?
(a) narcotic administration
(b) maternal exhaustion
(c) fetal malposition
(d) multiparity

5. Factors that increase the risk of umbilical cord prolapse include all of the following *except:*
(a) hydramnios
(b) fetal engagement
(c) more than one fetus
(d) a transverse lie

6. When umbilical cord prolapse occurs, rapid assessment and intervention by the health care team can help the client and fetus survive this traumatic event. Which of the following actions is *not* advised in this emergency situation? Explain your answer.
(a) Attempt to reinsert the cord if it protrudes from the vagina.
(b) Immediately summon help to prepare for a prompt delivery or surgery.
(c) Place the client in a knee-chest or Trendelenburg position.
(d) Prepare to administer oxygen by face mask and I.V. fluids.

Study questions

7. List three potential fetal effects of dysfunctional labor.

8. Describe some appropriate nursing actions to take when a client experiences uterine inversion during delivery of the placenta.

9. When precipitate labor occurs, the nurse may be the only health care professional who attends the delivery. What are some general nursing responsibilities in this case?

10. What is the cardinal sign of placenta previa?

11. Identify at least four conditions that may contribute to abruptio placentae.

12. List three signs of fetal distress.

13. Describe at least five actions the nurse should take in response to fetal distress; provide rationales for each action.

14. Unexpected intrapartal complications, such as placenta previa, can cause alarm in the client and family, leading to a nursing diagnosis of *anxiety related to uncertain perinatal outcome.* Discuss the role the nurse plays during this crisis to meet the client's and family's emotional needs.

Fill in the blank

15. Uterine dysfunction is classified as either ____________ or ____________ .

16. Precipitate labor is characterized by rapid __________ and typically lasts less than __________ hours.

17. In the condition called __________, the placenta has an abnormally low implantation, forming near or over the cervical os.

18. Premature placental separation after 20 weeks' gestation is known as __________.

19. Normally, amniotic fluid volume at term measures approximately __________ ml; when it exceeds 2,000 ml, the condition called __________ exists.

20. The most common fetal malpresentation is __________ presentation.

◆ CHAPTER 34 ◆

NEONATAL ADAPTATION

CHAPTER OVERVIEW

To survive, the neonate must assume the life-support functions previously performed by the placenta. Birth begins a transitional period—a critical and complex 24-hour phase during which the neonate must adjust from intrauterine to extrauterine life. The nurse who is familiar with the events of the transitional period can help ensure a successful adjustment, detecting deviations from the normal progression of neonatal adaptation and intervening promptly if such deviations occur. Chapter 34 helps prepare the nurse to work with neonates during the transitional period. It reviews the biological characteristics of neonatal adaptation during this time, discussing the major changes occurring in each body system. It describes the behavioral characteristics of adaptation, including neonatal sensory capacities and responses to environmental stimulation. The chapter concludes by exploring the periods of neonatal reactivity and neonatal sleep-awake patterns.

STUDENT ACTIVITIES

To test your familiarity with the information in this chapter, complete the following activities.

Clinical simulations

1. Robin Mardsley, a primiparous client, and her husband Richard are getting acquainted with their newborn son in the delivery room. When they notice that his hands and feet appear blue, they become alarmed and ask the nurse if this means he is having trouble breathing. What is the name for the condition that the Mardsleys have noticed? The nurse should provide what explanation for this condition?

2. Blanche Althus, age 30, asks the nurse about the blood she found on her newborn daughter's diaper this morning, 1 day after delivery. She also expresses concern that her daughter has swollen breasts and that a watery fluid leaked from the left breast several hours earlier. She says these problems did not occur with her firstborn, a boy. How should the nurse respond?

3. Sixteen hours after Liz Irwin delivers her daughter Brittany, the pediatrician informs her that Brittany has developed jaundice and has an unconjugated serum bilirubin level of 14 mg/dl. Which form of jaundice does the pediatrician diagnose? What conditions can cause this form of jaundice? Identify some problems Brittany may experience if she is not treated.

4. Tanya Zanelli, age 17, is a primiparous client who wishes to breast-feed her neonate. After an uneventful labor and delivery, she asks the nurse if she can begin breast-feeding in the delivery room. She states that she knows her son is hungry because he is sucking on his fist. Should the nurse encourage or discourage her to breast-feed at this time? Explain your answer.

Multiple choice

5. Adequate surfactant in the neonate's lungs at birth does *not:*
   (a) facilitate gas exchange
   (b) decrease inflation pressures needed to open the airways
   (c) increase the labor of breathing
   (d) improve lung co mpliance

6. What is the strongest stimulus for the neonate's first breath?
   (a) thermal changes
   (b) asphyxia
   (c) tactile stimulation
   (d) mechanical compression

7. Which of the following is *not* a major defense against neonatal heat loss? Explain your answer.
   (a) vasomotor control
   (b) thermal insulation
   (c) muscle activity
   (d) shivering

8. Which body system does *not* participate directly in neonatal bilirubin clearance?
   (a) respiratory system
   (b) hepatic system
   (c) renal system
   (d) gastrointestinal system

Study questions

9. What is the difference between functional and anatomic closure of the foramen ovale?

10. For the neonate to assume independent ventilation and oxygenation, fluid must be replaced by air in the respiratory tract at birth. Describe the three mechanical forces that lead to fluid removal from the neonate's lungs during vaginal delivery.

11. List four conditions necessary to maintain neonatal respiratory function within the first 24 hours after delivery.

12. Why is the neonate at risk for hemorrhage for several days after birth? Which treatment is used to prevent neonatal hemorrhage?

13. Identify the complex functions performed by the neonate's neurologic system to regulate adaptation during the transitional period.

14. List four categories of basic neonatal reflexes that are crucial to survival and must be present at birth.

15. Describe the four mechanisms of neonatal heat loss; for each mechanism, provide a nursing action that helps prevents significant cooling.

16. Why does the neonate lose 5% to 15% of the birth weight during the first 5 days after delivery?

17. Briefly describe the full range of neonatal sensory capacities, and explain how these capacities help the neonate adapt to the extrauterine environment.

18. The neonate's initial hours are marked by a series of behavioral and physiologic characteristics. What is this series called? How can familiarity with this series help the nurse enhance neonatal care?

19. Which period of reactivity is optimal for early mother-infant bonding? How long does this period last, and which characteristics does the neonate demonstrate during this period?

20. Identify conditions that can lead to hypoglycemia in the normal neonate.

21. Which nerve pathways are the first to develop in the neonate? What functions do these pathways serve?

Fill in the blank

22. Inadequate lung fluid removal in the neonate may lead to a respiratory disorder called ____________.

23. The neonate's most efficient heat production mechanism is ____________. In this mechanism, heat is produced through lipolysis of ____________.

(Continued on next page)

Identifying anatomic structures

24. On the illustrations below, identify the sites of functional closure of the three fetal structures and trace the circulation to show how blood ultimately flows to the neonate's liver and lungs.

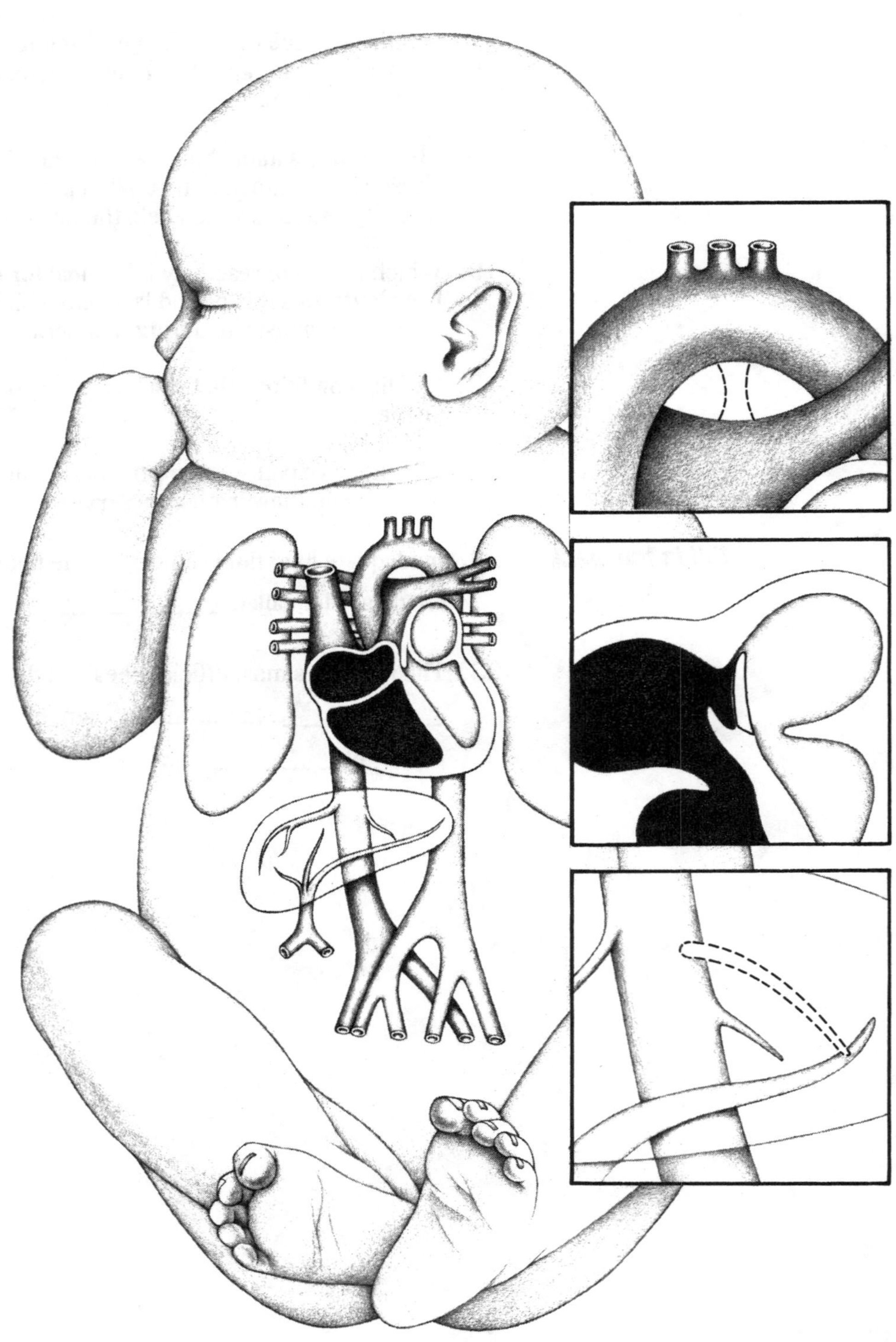

◆ CHAPTER 35 ◆

NEONATAL ASSESSMENT

CHAPTER OVERVIEW

During the first few days after delivery, the neonate must undergo thorough, systematic examinations to establish a baseline for comparison and to determine the adequacy of the transition to the extrauterine environment. Besides possessing the clinical skills for neonatal assessment, the nurse must understand the significance of assessment findings to identify potential or actual problems promptly. Chapter 35 provides a conceptual framework for neonatal assessment. It presents general assessment guidelines, describing the proper timing and sequence of the various types of assessment and explaining how periods of neonatal reactivity may affect findings. After delineating the steps of the brief physical assessment, it discusses gestational-age assessment, exploring the link between gestational-age and birth-weight variations and certain perinatal problems. Then it reviews the components of the complete physical assessment, identifying normal and abnormal findings. The chapter concludes by discussing the behavioral assessment.

STUDENT ACTIVITIES

To test your familiarity with the information in this chapter, complete the following activities.

Clinical simulations

1. Mimi Warren, age 16, delivered her daughter Beth at 37 weeks' gestation, based on the date of her last menstrual period (LMP). After completing a gestational-age assessment and plotting the findings on the Colorado intrauterine growth chart, the nurse determines that Beth is large for gestational age (LGA). Define this birth-weight variation, and briefly discuss the antepartal history findings that might have predicted it.

2. At delivery, Janis Riordan's newborn daughter Katy has Apgar scores of 7 and 10; she requires only bulb suctioning and a few whiffs of oxygen. Calculation by LMP suggests that Katy is preterm, born at 36 weeks' gestation. The nurse examines Katy and finds that she appears alert and active, without acute distress, and has no apparent congenital defects. She weighs 2,050 g and measures 42 cm in length and 29 cm in head circumference. Ten hours after delivery, the nurse assesses Katy's gestational age using the Ballard tool, with the results shown below.

Physical maturity findings

- skin: superficial peeling and a few visible veins
- lanugo: thinning on the back
- plantar surface: creases covering the entire sole
- breast: raised areola; breast bud measures 4 mm

- eye and ear: soft, curved pinna that recoils readily
- genitalia: labia majora larger than labia minora, but labia minora clearly visible

Neuromuscular maturity findings
- posture: legs and arms loosely flexed
- square window: 30 degrees
- arm recoil: less than 90 degrees
- popliteal angle: 90 degrees
- scarf sign: elbow just reaches midline
- heel to ear: heel does not rise above hip

Determine Katy's gestational age according to the Ballard tool (text pages 842 and 843). Then find her gestational-age and birth-weight classifications by plotting her gestational age and weight on the Colorado intrauterine growth chart (text page 840). Using Katy's case as an example, discuss the importance of plotting weight and gestational age on the growth chart.

Multiple choice

3. Which general guideline does *not* apply when performing a comprehensive neonatal assessment? Explain your answer.
(a) Adapt the assessment to the neonate's tolerance level to conserve the neonate's energy.
(b) Be organized and systematic and maintain a neutral thermal environment.
(c) Perform each component of all assessment tools—even if this results in duplication—to allow comparison and replicate the accuracy of findings.
(d) Allow the neonate to sleep undisturbed if sleep occurs during the assessment.

4. A bulging anterior fontanel typically signifies:
(a) dehydration
(b) premature closure of cranial sutures
(c) increased intracranial pressure
(d) normal scalp swelling after a difficult delivery

5. A positive Ortolani's maneuver indicates:
(a) hydrocephalus
(b) neurologic dysfunction
(c) birth injury
(d) congenital hip dislocation

6. If neonatal assessment reveals several of Smith's minor abnormalities, the nurse should suspect:
(a) birth injury
(b) major congenital anomalies
(c) an abdominal tumor
(d) a patent ductus arteriosus

Study questions

7. Explain why the nurse should review the maternal antepartal and intrapartal records when a neonate is admitted to the nursery.

8. Identify the five components of the immediate neonatal assessment.

9. Why must the nurse consider the specific period of neonatal reactivity when performing the physical and behavioral assessments?

10. The following are typical vital sign measurements obtained for neonates during the first 2 hours after delivery. After each finding, state whether it is normal or abnormal; if a finding is abnormal, provide some possible causes.
   (a) Pulse—140 beats/minute: ___N___
   (b) Respiratory rate—70 breaths/minute: ___AB___ N - 40-70/min
   (c) Axillary temperature—95.8° F: ___AB___
   (d) Blood pressure—66/40 mm Hg: ___N___
   (e) Respiratory rate—44 breaths/minute: ___N___
   (f) Rectal temperature—99.2° F: ___N___

(36.5-37; 97.7-99)

11. What are some signs of labored breathing that the nurse might detect when assessing a neonate's respiratory pattern?

12. Discuss the two most commonly used gestational-age assessment tools, and cite the major differences between them.

13. Briefly describe cephalhematoma and caput succedaneum.

14. The chart below shows normal responses to neonatal reflexes. In the blanks in the appropriate columns, place the name of each reflex and briefly describe the testing method.

NORMAL RESPONSE	REFLEX	TESTING METHOD
a. Neonates extends extremities on the side to which the head is turned and flexes extremities on the opposite side.		
b. Neonate makes walking motions with both feet.		
c. Neonate extends and abducts all extremities bilaterally and symmetically; forms a "C" shape with the thumb and forefinger; and adducts then reflexes, extremities.		
d. Neonate sucks on a finger forcefully and rhythmically; sucking is coordinated with swallowing.		
e. Neonate hyperextends the toes, dorsiflexes the great toe, and fans the toes outward.		

15. Identify the six categories of behavioral responses evaluated on the Brazelton neonatal behavioral assessment scale.

16. Why should the nurse encourage parents to observe the behavioral assessment of their neonate?

Fill in the blank

17. When taking a neonate's anthropometric measurements, the nurse should expect chest circumference to measure __________ cm less than head circumference.

18. A neonate's crown-to-rump length should approximate the circumference of the __________ .

19. Gestational-age assessment tools evaluate external physical features and __________ maturity rather than birth weight as indices of growth and maturation.

20. For the term neonate, average length is __________ cm; head circumference typically measures __________ cm.

Matching terms and definitions

21. Match each description in the left column with the corresponding neonatal skin variation in the right column.

(1) deep pink, flat, localized areas of capillary dilation, typically seen on the upper eyelids, nasal bridge, and occipital bone	(a) Mongolian spots
(2) pink, papular rash covering the thorax, back, abdomen, and groin; commonly appears within 24 to 48 hours after birth	(b) cutaneous papilloma
(3) small brownish or flesh-colored outgrowth of skin, possibly signifying congenital anomaly	(c) telangiectatic nevi
(4) color division at midline	(d) café-au-lait spots
(5) permanent birthmark; a flat, capillary hemangioma ranging from pale red to deep purple	(e) harlequin sign
(6) minute white epidermal cysts caused by sebaceous gland obstruction; commonly seen on the face	(f) milia

(7) blue-black macule over the buttocks, possibly extending to the sacral region	(g) miliaria
(8) rash consisting of minute vesicles and papules, seen mainly on the forehead and in skinfolds	(h) erythema toxicum
(9) light tan macules that may indicate neurofibromatosis	(i) nevus flammeus

◆ CHAPTER 36 ◆

NURSING CARE OF THE NORMAL NEONATE

CHAPTER OVERVIEW

Chapter 36 describes the nurse's role in promoting successful neonatal adaptation, family adjustment to the neonate, and optimal parent-infant interaction. It describes how the nurse helps maintain the neonate's physiologic stability by ensuring adequate thermoregulation, oxygenation, hydration, nutrition, elimination, and hygiene. Detailing ongoing assessment, the chapter explains how to prevent and assess neonatal complications. It discusses how to plan and implement nursing care for the normal neonate, elaborating on routine neonatal care measures and environmental safety. The chapter examines the cultural factors that may influence parental attitudes toward circumcision and details parent teaching and discharge planning. To ease the neonate's adjustment to the home and foster parent-infant bonding, it emphasizes a family-centered approach.

STUDENT ACTIVITIES

To test your familiarity with the information in this chapter, complete the following activities.

Clinical simulations

1. Several hours after Nancy Miner, a primiparous client, delivers her son Jason, she calls the nursery to find out when Jason can visit with her again. To determine whether Jason's body temperature has stabilized adequately to allow such a visit, the nurse should follow what guidelines?

2. Treena Cernuka, age 28, asks the nurse when she can begin bottle-feeding her daughter Emily, who is almost 6 hours old. Is an initial feeding appropriate at this time? How should the nurse assess Emily during and after the initial feeding?

3. Carla Dunbar is being prepared for discharge 1 day after delivering her son Steven, whom she is breast-feeding. To help Ms. Dunbar ensure that Steven receives adequate hydration and has a normal urinary elimination pattern, the nurse should provide what teaching?

4. Stephanie Briggs, a nurse educator, is planning a class on environmental home safety for postpartal clients. Identify some neonatal safety measures she should include.

Multiple choice

5. In a neonate, abdominal distention, a persistent and pronounced rise or drop in the heart or respiratory rate, lethargy during periods of expected activity, and temperature instability represent:
   (a) normal baseline fluctuations
   (b) transient changes during a specific period of neonatal reactivity
   (c) distress
   (d) expected alterations during an initial bath.

6. The narrow temperature range that maintains a stable core temperature with minimal caloric and oxygen consumption is called:
   (a) hyperthermia
   (b) a neutral thermal environment
   (c) thermogenesis
   (d) ambient temperature regulation

7. Which of the following findings does *not* signify cold stress in a neonate?
   (a) hypercalcemia
   (b) an accelerated respiratory rate
   (c) labored respirations
   (d) hypoglycemia

Study questions

8. Identify seven factors that the nurse must evaluate continually to detect neonatal instability.

9. When caring for a neonate during the first few days after delivery, the nurse must be prepared to suction the airway to prevent mucus aspiration and maintain oxygenation. Explain why a bulb syringe is preferred over a sterile suction catheter for this procedure.

10. For the first few hours after delivery, the nurse must stay alert for changes in the neonate's respiratory pattern that may signal respiratory distress. What are these signs?

11. Describe the appearance and progression of neonatal bowel movements, and compare and contrast the bowel elimination patterns of breast-fed and formula-fed neonates during the first week after delivery.

12. Because the neonate lacks localized immune reactions, infection causes only subtle, nonspecific signs. List at least five nonspecific signs that suggest neonatal infection.

13. Discuss an appropriate role for the nurse when teaching parents how to provide neonatal care. Also, explain how rooming-in of the neonate can enhance parental caregiving skills.

14. Identify three factors that may influence the parents' attitude toward circumcision.

◆ CHAPTER 37 ◆

INFANT NUTRITION

CHAPTER OVERVIEW

The infant's rapid growth and development during the first year necessitate optimal nutrition. Besides contributing to infant health, nutrition enhances parent-infant bonding and provides important social interactions. Chapter 37 prepares the nurse to promote optimal infant nutrition. It describes nutrient and fluid requirements and special nutritional limitations for neonates and infants. After discussing breast-feeding and formula-feeding, it examines the factors that influence the parents' choice of infant feeding method. It describes the physiology of lactation, breast milk composition, and infant sucking dynamics during breast-feeding, then provides basic information about formula feeding. Next, the chapter discusses nursing care related to infant nutrition. It explains how to assess a breast-feeding client's knowledge of feeding techniques, then tells how to evaluate a client's knowledge of formula-feeding techniques and infant formula intake requirements. The chapter concludes with nursing interventions for both breast-feeding and formula-feeding clients, emphasizing client teaching.

STUDENT ACTIVITIES

To test your familiarity with the information in this chapter, complete the following activities.

Clinical simulations

1. Amy Barnes, a primiparous client age 22, has just delivered a healthy, full-term daughter after an uncomplicated labor without medication. During repair of her episiotomy, she asks the nurse if she can begin breast-feeding her daughter. Is this a good idea? Explain your answer.

2. Amy's husband Dave asks the nurse what support he can provide to enhance Amy's breast-feeding after her discharge. The nurse should offer what guidance?

3. When Amy asks how she can tell if her daughter is getting enough milk from breast-feeding, the nurse should provide which general guidelines?

4. Amy mentions that her sister gave supplementary bottles of formula to her neonate after the first week of breast-feeding. Should the nurse encourage Amy to follow suit?

5. During a postpartal home visit to Elise Johnson, a primiparous client age 19, the public health nurse discovers that Ms. Johnson has been feeding whole cow's milk to her 2-week-old son. Ms. Johnson

explains that she has a limited budget. "That fancy formula seemed too expensive when milk in the grocery store is just as good," she says. How should the nurse respond?

6. Ms. Johnson asks the nurse when she can start adding cereal to her son's bottle. She says her mother is encouraging her to do this because "it will help him sleep through the night." How should the nurse respond?

7. Sherry Ettinger, a new adolescent mother, plans to feed her neonate formula. When evaluating Ms. Ettinger during the immediate postpartal period, the nurse should assess which maternal and neonatal factors related to formula-feeding?

8. Briefly identify the factors the nurse should evaluate when observing Jane Poirier, a primiparous client, as she breast-feeds her neonate during the early postpartal period.

9. Donna Morasco, a primiparous client age 21, plans to feed her newborn son infant formula. When teaching her how to burp her son, the nurse should demonstrate which positions and should provide what related information?

10. How can the nurse help Ms. Morasco establish a feeding pattern?

Multiple choice

11. Which of the following is *not* a characteristic of women who are able to breast-feed for prolonged periods? Explain your answer.
(a) They provide more frequent feedings in the early days at home.
(b) They show a greater ability to relax.
(c) They are better able to isolate themselves from the demands of other children during breast-feeding.
(d) They receive more support from their partner.

12. Lactation insufficiency usually results from:
(a) psychological factors
(b) mismanagement of lactation
(c) fatigue and depression
(d) breast engorgement

Study questions

13. List the three basic nutrients that supply the infant's caloric needs, and briefly describe their physiologic functions.

14. Briefly describe the changes in breast milk composition over the course of a feeding.

15. What are the signs of lactose intolerance in the neonate? Identify the cause of this disorder, and name a common treatment.

16. When providing teaching for a client planning to breast-feed, the nurse should include which topics?

17. Identify the four basic methods of infant formula preparation.

18. Briefly discuss the components and benefits of colostrum.

19. When do infant growth spurts occur?

Fill in the blank

20. The neonate needs ___________ ml of fluid per kg/day, compared to 20 to 30 ml per kg/day needed by the adult.

21. The three major indices used to assess an infant's nutritional status are ___________ , ___________ , and ___________ .

22. Birth weight typically doubles by age 5 to 6 months and triples by age ___________ .

23. Daily infant formula intake should average _________ ml/kg.

Chronological order

24. Each statement below describes a physiologic event occurring during the let-down reflex, which makes breast milk available to the infant. Indicate the correct chronological order of these events by placing a number from 1 to 5 next to each statement.
(a) Myoepithelial cells surrounding the alveoli contract.
(b) Milk is available through nipple openings.
(c) The hypothalamus triggers release of oxytocin by the posterior pituitary gland.
(d) Milk is ejected into the ductules and sinuses.
(e) Nipple stimulation or an emotional response to the infant occurs.

Matching related elements

25. Match the appropriate infant feeding method in the left column with the health benefit described in the right column. (Each feeding method has more than one benefit.)

(1) breast-feeding	(a) promotes immunologic defenses through antibody transfer
(2) formula-feeding	(b) requires preparation, refrigeration, and storage
	(c) may enhance mother-infant bonding
	(d) lengthens the interval between feedings
	(e) avoids the potential need to restrict the mother's diet or medications
	(f) is nutritionally superior
	(g) promotes development of facial muscles, jaws, and teeth

Values clarification

A nurse's personal feelings about infant feeding methods can influence a client's choice of feeding method—especially during client teaching. This exercise will help identify your feelings about infant feeding methods, increasing your awareness of any bias in the care or information you provide clients. Complete each of the following statements with the first thought that comes to mind.

26. I believe that the simplest, most convenient, and most beneficial infant feeding method is.....

27. If a client had problems getting a fussy neonate to attach to her breast, I would feel ...

28. Teaching postpartal clients about formula preparation and proper care of the equipment would make me feel ...

29. I believe the use of supplementary bottles for the inexperienced breast-feeding client is ...

30. One piece of advice I would give to all breast-feeding women is ...

31. When it comes to formula feeding, I feel that new mothers should ...

32. The one instance in which I would discourage a new mother from choosing a particular infant feeding method is when ...

What did this exercise teach you? If it revealed a bias toward or against a particular feeding method, you must devise a way to present information objectively when working with expectant and postpartal clients.

◆ CHAPTER 38 ◆

HIGH-RISK NEONATES

CHAPTER OVERVIEW

High-risk neonates—those with an increased risk of death or chronic disability during the perinatal period—require prompt medical intervention before or shortly after delivery to ensure an optimal outcome. As maternal and fetal medicine become more highly advanced, the number of high-risk neonates increases. The challenge of perinatal nursing care is to ensure survival for these neonates while minimizing long-term sequelae.

Chapter 38 discusses the nurse's role in caring for high-risk neonates. It examines regionalization of perinatal care and discusses key ethical and legal concerns. Then it describes the etiology and pathophysiology of perinatal problems that lead to high-risk status, highlighting gestational-age and birth-weight variations. Next, the chapter presents nursing care for the high-risk neonate. It explores the factors that help predict high-risk status and explains how to assess for each perinatal problem described earlier. Then the chapter describes nursing interventions, focusing on emergency measures and resuscitation drugs. It delineates general nursing interventions, including measures that support oxygenation, thermoregulation, and nutrition. The chapter concludes by describing some special procedures and outlining medical and nursing management of selected perinatal problems.

STUDENT ACTIVITIES

To test your familiarity with the information in this chapter, complete the following activities.

Clinical simulations

1. During the second trimester of pregnancy, Cathy Graham, age 28, is diagnosed with gestational diabetes. At 36 weeks' gestation, her son Bennett is born by cesarean delivery; at 9 lb, 2 oz, he is large for gestational age (LGA). What potential perinatal complications does Bennett face besides those related to his gestational-age and birth-weight variations?

2. When assessing Bennett for hypoglycemia, the nurse should stay alert for which signs? How is the diagnosis of hypoglycemia confirmed?

3. Jonathan Rubin, born at 32 weeks' gestation, is diagnosed with erythroblastosis fetalis. His treatment plan includes phototherapy and exchange transfusions. Describe the general focus of nursing measures during phototherapy, and identify specific nursing actions that will help ensure his safety during this treatment.

4. Althea Maxon, age 24, delivers her daughter Maura at 35 weeks' gestation after smoking crack cocaine. She admits to using I.V. drugs while pregnant and states that fear of legal ramifications kept her from seeking prenatal care. Because of Ms. Maxon's history of drug use, the physician orders a human immunodeficiency virus (HIV) test for Maura. The nurse should assess Maura for which signs of HIV infection?

Multiple choice

5. Regionalized perinatal helps ensure the highest quality of care by:
(a) reducing the need for transport to another facility, thereby fostering bonding between parents and their high-risk neonate
(b) guaranteeing that all facilities have at least the minimum equipment and staff needed to care for unanticipated high-risk neonates
(c) eliminating the need for all health care facilities to acquire the advanced technology and staff for a neonatal intensive care unit (NICU)
(d) improving the resources within each facility through continuing education and grant funding for equipment

6. According to guidelines established by the American Academy of Pediatrics and the American College of Obstetricians and Gynecologists, a neonate born at 35 weeks' gestation with moderate respiratory distress syndrome should receive treatment at a:
(a) level 1, 2, or 3 perinatal care facility
(b) level 2 perinatal care facility only
(c) level 3 perinatal care facility only
(d) level 2 or 3 perinatal care facility

7. Which of the following is *not* a major focus of a level 3 perinatal center?
(a) client and community education
(b) research and outcome surveillance
(c) graduate and postgraduate education
(d) system management

Study questions

8. State the three major goals of neonatal intensive care.

9. Briefly discuss the ethical issues that may arise when a neonate is born with meningomyelocele.

10. What are the three most common problems seen in the NICU?

11. Identify the complications that may arise in a neonate with prolonged asphyxia.

12. List at least six congenital anomalies that pose a threat to the neonate's life and warrant immediate intervention.

13. For each description below, name the congenital heart defect to which it applies.
(a) Abnormal opening between the pulmonary artery and the aorta resulting from failure of the fetal circulatory structure to close after delivery; allows blood to shunt from the aorta to the pulmonary artery

(b) Anomaly consisting of four defects; may result in such hemodynamic changes as a left-to-right or a right-to-left shunt (which allows unoxygenated blood from the right ventricle to enter the aorta directly)
(c) Abnormal opening in the atrial septum that allows blood to shunt from the left to right atrium, causing enlargement of the right ventricle and atrium
(d) Defect in which the pulmonary and systemic circulations cannot mix due to abnormal origins of the pulmonary artery and aorta
(e) Anomaly in which obstructed preductal or postductal blood flow causes pressure in the left ventricle to rise; compensatory collateral circulation enhances blood flow from the proximal arteries and bypasses the obstructed areas

14. Identify six measures used to resuscitate a neonate immediately after delivery.

15. How can the nurse promote parent-infant bonding during a neonate's extended stay in the NICU?

16. Various factors can cause fluid imbalance in the high-risk neonate. To ensure high-quality care, the nurse must be able to recognize signs of both fluid volume deficit and fluid volume excess. The clinical findings listed below are important indices of neonatal fluid status. Which findings reflect fluid volume excess? Which reflect fluid volume deficit?
(a) edema
(b) poor skin turgor
(c) low-grade fever
(d) rhonchi
(e) elevated hematocrit
(f) dyspnea
(g) sunken fontanels
(h) increasing central venous pressure
(i) urine output of 7 ml/kg/hr

Fill in the blank

17. A preterm neonate is one born before completion of week ___________ of gestation.

18. A postterm neonate is one born after completion of week ___________ of gestation.

19. A small-for-gestational-age (SGA) neonate is one whose birth weight falls below the ___________ percentile for gestational age.

20. A large-for-gestational-age (LGA) neonate is one whose birth weight exceeds the ___________ percentile for gestational age.

True or false

21. The neonatal mortality rate refers to the number of deaths per 10,000 live births within the first 28 days after delivery.
❑ True ❑ False

22. The neonate with a low birth weight is twice as likely to die within 1 month after delivery than one with an average birth weight.
❑ True ❑ False

23. The two most common congenital musculoskeletal anomalies are congenital hip dislocation and talipes (clubfoot).
❑ True ❑ False

Chronological order

24. The American Heart Association and American Academy of Pediatrics have established guidelines for immediate resuscitation of the neonate with cardiopulmonary compromise. Some basic steps of this protocol are shown below. Arrange the steps in the order in which they should be performed by placing a number from 1 to 9 next to each statement.
(a) Assess the heart rate.
(b) Place the neonate under a radiant warmer.
(c) If the heart rate is below 60 beats/minute, begin cardiac massage.
(d) Suction the neonate's mouth, then nose.
(e) Assess respirations.
(f) If the heart rate above is 100 beats/minute and the neonate is breathing regularly, provide gentle stimulation.
(g) Dry the neonate.
(h) respirations are not spontaneous, begin positive-pressure ventilation with a bag and mask.

Matching terms and definitions

25. Match each gestational-age and birth-weight classification shown in the left column with the associated perinatal problems in the right column. (Some perinatal problems are associated with more than one classification.)

(1) preterm	(a) hyperbilirubinemia
(2) postterm	(b) infection
(3) SGA	(c) asphyxia
(4) LGA	(d) polycythemia
	(e) intraventricular hemorrhage
	(f) respiratory distress syndrome
	(g) birth trauma
	(h) asymmetric organ development
	(i) patent ductus arteriosus

(j) learning disabilities

(k) hypoglycemia

(1) congenital anomalies

(m) hypocalcemia

(n) retinopathy

(o) meconium aspiration

(p) bronchopulmonary dysplasia

◆ CHAPTER 39 ◆

CARE OF THE FAMILIES OF HIGH-RISK NEONATES

CHAPTER OVERVIEW

When a fetus or neonate does not survive or has a problem that entails lengthy hospitalization or chronic disability, the family experiences grief and loss. During this crisis, nursing care must address the family's psychological needs as well as the neonate's physical needs. The nurse can help the family cope by encouraging them to seek out support systems or resources that provide ongoing assistance, teaching them about the neonate's condition and future care, and maintaining empathetic contact with them as they work to integrate the high-risk neonate into family life. Chapter 39 describes family reactions to the birth of a high-risk neonate, defines the functions and dimensions of grief, and explores variations in grief expression associated with circumstances or cultural influences. It applies the nursing process to care of the families of high-risk neonates, highlighting nursing interventions that promote parent-infant bonding.

STUDENT ACTIVITIES

To test your familiarity with the information in this chapter, complete the following activities.

Clinical simulations

1. Carmelita Ayer, age 24, is a primigravid client in good health who has received regular prenatal care and has had no antepartal complications. She became pregnant 1 year after immigrating to the United States from Costa Rica; she and her husband Jorge have awaited the birth of their first child with much excitement.
   At term, after an uncomplicated 7-hour labor, Carmelita delivers a 5-lb, 3-oz daughter, Ana. Immediately, however, Ana shows evidence of chronic intrauterine hypoxia; she then develops meconium aspiration syndrome and is transferred to a neonatal intensive care unit (NICU) in serious condition.

   For the first few weeks, Carmelita and Jorge visit Ana in the NICU regularly and assure their families in Costa Rica that she will be fine. Despite increasing evidence that Ana is not in stable condition—and despite her continuing need for intensive therapy—the Ayers believe that her hospitalization is just a minor setback. The nurse becomes increasingly concerned because they seem unwilling to accept the reality and seriousness of Ana's condition.

   What coping mechanism best describes the Ayers' reaction to the crisis created by Ana's critical illness? Explain why their reaction concerns the perinatal team caring for Ana.

2. On several occasions, the nurse sees Carmelita stroking Ana tearfully, reassuring her that her mother is with her. Jorge, in contrast, seems distant and uninvolved. In a perinatal team conference, the nurse notes that Carmelita's response to Ana's worsening condition seems more appropriate than Jorge's.
Identify some cultural customs that may be affecting Jorge's expression of grief, and explain why the nurse must consider these customs when evaluating his behavior.

3. During one of the Ayers' visits to the NICU, the nurse asks them if they have any health-related cultural or religious customs they wish to incorporate into Ana's care. Explain the purpose of this question.

4. Unfortunately, Ana's condition does not improve. After 28 days in the NICU, her death appears imminent. To help Carmelita and Jorge deal with their impending loss, the nurse should implement which interventions?

5. Shortly after an uneventful labor and delivery, Josie and Mike Greene, a couple in their mid-thirties, learn that their neonate Patrick has been diagnosed with Down's syndrome and a cardiac defect that will require surgery within 1 year. Should the nurse expect the Greenes to achieve complete resolution of their grief before Josie's discharge? Explain your answer.

6. Describe two interventions the nurse can implement to enhance the support that the Greenes normally provide to each other.

7. Two weeks after Patrick Greene's birth, his brother Kevin, age 4, begins to have nightmares and habitually runs to his parents' bedroom in the middle of the night seeking comfort. The Greenes find this disruptive, especially after the long days they have been spending with Patrick as he is evaluated for his disabilities and prospective surgery. What problems may Kevin experience if his needs go unmet? How can the nurse help Kevin cope with the family crisis?

8. Margery Newkirk, a primigravid client with severe preeclampsia, has an emergency cesarean delivery at 32 weeks' gestation. Her daughter Regina is admitted to the NICU weighing 1,400 g. Margery's parents—Regina's grandparents—remain in the NICU waiting area to learn of their granddaughter's condition while Margery recovers from preeclampsia and surgery. Explain why the NICU nurse should be sensitive to the grandparents' unique needs.

Study questions

9. Identify the stages of grief as described by Kübler-Ross.

10. What are the dimensions of grief proposed individually by Bowlby, Parkes, and Davidson?

11. Describe how the family of a high-risk neonate may move through the stages of grief.

12. When a neonate is admitted to the NICU, the nurse should include which factors in the initial assessment of the parents?

13. Which support systems do parents of high-risk neonates use most actively? What other potential sources of support might parents rely on?

14. Identify four general nursing interventions for the family of a high-risk neonate.

15. When evaluating the parents' ability and motivation to assume primary care for a high-risk neonate, the nurse should assess for which specific behaviors to determine whether they need further nursing intervention before the neonate's discharge?

16. Describe four ways in which the nurse can involve the parents in the care of a high-risk neonate to improve their parenting skills and enhance parent-infant bonding.

◆ CHAPTER 40 ◆

DISCHARGE PLANNING AND NEONATAL CARE AT HOME

CHAPTER OVERVIEW

The rising incidence of high-risk neonates and the trend toward early discharge of healthy neonates have increased the demand for home health care services. Chapter 40 discusses the nurse's role in discharge planning and home health care for neonates. First, it describes discharge planning systems and resources and explains how to identify the specific discharge planning needs of a neonate and family. Then it tells how the nurse implements the discharge plan by preparing the parents for the neonate's discharge. The chapter describes home health care services, equipment, and supplies, identifying the types of home health care a neonate may need. It explains how to evaluate parental knowledge, caregiving skills, and support needs for the neonate receiving care at home; how to assess whether health care can be delivered safely and adequately in the home; and how to gauge parent-infant interaction. Then it discusses such nursing interventions as ensuring parental caregiving knowledge and skills and promoting parent-infant interaction.

STUDENT ACTIVITIES

To test your familiarity with the information in this chapter, complete the following activities.

Clinical simulations

1. Scott Harris, delivered at 33 weeks' gestation, requires a lengthy hospitalization for complications related to prematurity—including severe respiratory distress syndrome and hyperbilirubinemia. Finally, he is weaned from the mechanical ventilator and prepared for discharge. However, he will require home apnea monitoring. List at least six factors the nurse should assess to determine the discharge planning needs of Dawn and Peter, Scott's parents.

2. What knowledge and skills must the Harrises possess to provide proper care for Scott at home during apnea monitoring?

3. Kevin Moletierre, age 3 weeks, has been diagnosed with acquired immunodeficiency syndrome (AIDS)—the result of transplacental infection. Identify the parental factors the nurse should assess when preparing for his discharge.

Study questions

4. At what point in a neonate's hospitalization should discharge planning begin?

5. Identify the nurse's four major discharge planning responsibilities, as defined in the standards of neonatal nursing developed by NAACOG, the organization for obstetric, gynecologic, and neonatal nurses.

6. Which in-facility resource personnel typically are involved in discharge planning?

7. Identify four possible alternatives to home care for neonates and infants who are ready for discharge but require continued medical care.

8. When preparing parents for a neonate's discharge, the nurse should include which teaching topics and use which teaching strategies?

9. When documenting the neonate's discharge plan on the medical record, the nurse must include which information, as stipulated by the Joint Commission on Accreditation of Healthcare Organizations?

10. In what circumstances is case management of a neonate's home health care most helpful?

11. Identify three benefits of home care for the ventilator-dependent neonate.

12. Explain why the nurse should become familiar with local parent support groups and refer parents of special-needs neonates to these groups when appropriate.

◆ CHAPTER 41 ◆

PHYSIOLOGY OF THE POSTPARTAL PERIOD

CHAPTER OVERVIEW

After delivery, the dramatic physiologic changes that accompany pregnancy reverse. Within approximately 6 weeks, all body systems have resumed nonpregnancy status, returning to normal physiologic functioning. To help the postpartal client recover optimal health and begin adjusting to life with her new neonate, the nurse must be familiar with the physical and emotional effects of this process. Chapter 41 provides the theoretical basis necessary for the nurse to promote resumption of normal body function in postpartal clients. It describes the significant anatomic and physiologic changes that follow delivery, emphasizing the reproductive and endocrine systems. The chapter then explains how other body systems resume normal anatomic and functional status.

STUDENT ACTIVITIES

To test your familiarity with the information in this chapter, complete the following activities.

Clinical simulations

1. On admission to the postpartal unit after delivering her second child, Mary-Grace Hannaberry, age 27, complains of discomfort similar to labor pains. She requests pain medication frequently and reports that the discomfort is worse immediately after she breast-feeds her neonate. She asks the nurse why she did not experience this discomfort after her first child and questions whether the pain is normal. How should the nurse respond?

2. During discharge preparation, the nurse informs Susan Stefani, a multigravid client age 29, that she should call the physician immediately if she experiences an abnormal lochial flow. How should the nurse describe the signs and symptoms of abnormal lochia?

3. Trina Fields, a primiparous client age 23, who is breast-feeding her neonate, has arrived for her 6-week postpartal follow-up appointment. She tells the nurse-midwife that her vagina feels dry and uncomfortable during intercourse, reports that she lacks interest in sex, and asks if sexual intercourse will ever feel "normal" to her again. How should the nurse-midwife respond?

4. During a class on postpartal adjustment, Greta Delaney, a multiparous client age 23, says she has heard that a breast-feeding woman cannot get pregnant until her menstrual period resumes and that

no woman can get pregnant until she has regular periods. She states that after her last child, her period did not resume until the infant began to wean at age 7 months. How should the nurse respond to Ms. Delaney's comments?

5. Michelle Saltz, a primiparous client age 32, is preparing for discharge from the postpartal unit. The nurse enters her room and finds her standing in front of a mirror inspecting her figure. Ms. Saltz explains that she had to send her husband home to bring a maternity dress because she could not fit into the other clothes he brought her. She asks the nurse why she still looks pregnant even though she delivered 2 days earlier. How should the nurse reply?

6. Jane Yarrow, age 36, describes extreme perspiration on the first night after delivery, when she awakened to find herself saturated. She tells the nurse she is concerned that she may have a fever or an infection. How should the nurse proceed?

7. When assessing Karen Beyer, a primiparous client, on the first day after delivery, where should the nurse expect to palpate the uterus?

Study questions

8. After delivery of the fetus and placenta, the uterus begins to return to a nonpregnant state. Which uterine structures are involved directly in this process?

9. Briefly describe the uterine mechanisms that cause uterine involution.

10. How long does the uterus take to regain a nonpregnant weight and size after delivery?

11. Define lochia and describe its stages.

12. Which three endocrine system structures coordinate the hormonal interaction that leads to postpartal resumption of the menstrual cycle? Which hormones are involved in this interaction?

13. Identify and discuss four mechanisms that help restore normal blood volume after delivery.

14. Why should the nurse discuss the danger signs of thrombophlebitis with postpartal clients during discharge preparation?

15. Explain why resumption of normal bowel motility is delayed after delivery.

16. The anatomic structures and body systems listed below undergo changes during pregnancy, delivery, or both. Briefly identify these changes and state the expected postpartal readjustment for each structure or system. Indicate whether the change is permanent (P) or temporary (T) next to each.

- uterus
- cervix
- breasts (in a nonlactating client)
- respiratory system
- cardiovascular system
- immune system
- integumentary system
- metabolic system

◆ CHAPTER 42 ◆

CARE DURING THE NORMAL POSTPARTAL PERIOD

CHAPTER OVERVIEW

Chapter 42 prepares the nurse to care for the postpartal client, helping to ensure her full recovery and promote the family's adjustment to the neonate. Delineating nursing assessment, the chapter describes ongoing evaluation of the client's vital signs, comfort level, rest and sleep patterns, psychosocial status, and body systems. It highlights assessment of the uterus and lochia and explains how to conduct a head-to-toe physical assessment. The chapter explores expected postpartal changes and discusses common deviations from the norm, explaining their significance. Then it presents nursing measures that promote uterine involution, reduce discomfort, and prevent postpartal complications. It highlights client teaching, including such topics as postpartal exercises and self-care after discharge.

STUDENT ACTIVITIES

To test your familiarity with the information in this chapter, complete the following activities.

Clinical simulations

1. After a 6-hour labor, Lucia Aguirre, age 24, delivers a 7-lb, 2-oz boy by normal vaginal delivery over an intact perineum. On her admission to the postpartal unit 2 hours later, the nurse reviews her labor and delivery records, which indicate that no complications occurred and that her blood loss approximated 250 ml. The nurse then performs a physical assessment, determining that Ms. Aguirre is in stable condition. Her fundus is firm and located at the umbilicus; she has scant lochia rubra. Her vital signs are as follows:

- temperature: 99.6° F
- pulse: 102 beats/minute
- respiratory rate: 22 breaths/minute
- blood pressure: 100/70 mm Hg

Ms. Aguirre is elated over the birth of her son and is eager to talk to her family about the birth experience. Although she complains of afterbirth pains, she has not requested pain medication; she has not been able to void since delivery. Which condition should the nurse suspect as the most likely cause of Ms. Aguirre's elevated temperature?

2. How should the nurse interpret Ms. Aguirre's pulse rate?

3. Describe some comfort measures the nurse might implement for Ms. Aguirre to reduce her afterbirth pains.

4. Tracey Neborsky, age 14, is a primigravid client who delivered a 6-lb daughter vaginally by vacuum extraction 4 hours ago after a long labor. On two separate occasions, the nurse measures her blood pressure at 140/98 mm Hg. Ms. Neborsky complains of a headache and blurred vision; her face and hands are swollen. How should the nurse proceed?

5. Patricia Jordan, a 38-year-old gravida 5, para 4014 client, had a 9-lb son 3 hours ago after an accelerated labor. During a postpartal assessment, the nurse determines that Ms. Jordan's uterus is soft and boggy. The nurse should suspect which condition as the cause of this finding?

6. Rosalie Kohan, age 34, is a primigravid client who delivered an 8-lb, 9-oz daughter by forceps over a right mediolateral episiotomy. Three hours after delivery, she still has not voided, despite her full bladder. Explain why the nurse should make every effort to have Ms. Kohan void spontaneously, and describe some appropriate nursing interventions.

7. During delivery, Martha Jenkins lost approximately 600 ml of blood. When assessing her on her admission to the postpartal unit, the nurse finds markedly elevated pulse and respiratory rates, decreased blood pressure, a firm fundus located at the midline, and bright red lochia flowing in a steady trickle. Explain why the nurse should suspect hemorrhage, and identify the most likely cause of hemorrhage in this case.

8. Nancy Farrell, who delivered vaginally over a mediolateral episiotomy 2 hours ago, complains of pain from her episiotomy stitches. Describe some appropriate measures the nurse should implement to increase Ms. Farrell's comfort and promote perineal healing.

9. Randi Cheng, a primigravid client age 31, complains of incisional pain and a pounding headache several hours after a cesarean delivery under spinal anesthesia. The nurse should suspect which condition as the cause of Ms. Cheng's symptoms? How should the nurse proceed?

Multiple choice

10. When given to a postpartal client, methylergonovine:
(a) has no effect
(b) may increase blood pressure
(c) may decrease blood pressure
(d) may cause wide swings in blood pressure

11. Which of the following is a normal postpartal assessment finding? Explain your answer.
(a) heavy vaginal bleeding, especially with clots and tissue fragments
(b) a temperature of 100.2° F or higher

(c) bilateral breast fullness and discomfort with nipple leakage
(d) a warm, red, tender area on a lower extremity

Study questions

12. List five signs of postpartal hemorrhage.

13. Describe normal perineal findings for the client with an episiotomy.

14. If a client does not void spontaneously within 6 to 8 hours after delivery, which intervention is necessary? Why?

15. When assessing the postpartal client, why must the nurse evaluate the lower extremities carefully? How should the nurse conduct this assessment?

16. Why is a client at risk for injury during the first few hours after delivery? To ensure client safety during this time, the nurse should take what steps?

17. Describe appropriate teaching for the client using the natural method of lactation suppression.

18. Identify some comfort measures for the postpartal client with hemorrhoids.

19. Which postpartal clients should receive Rh immune globulin (RhoGAM)? When should this preparation be administered?

20. Describe some teaching topics specific to multiparous postpartal clients.

21. Why is frequent respiratory assessment especially crucial for the client who had a caesarean delivery? What are the key components of this assessment?

◆ CHAPTER 43 ◆

PSYCHOSOCIAL ADAPTATION OF THE POSTPARTAL FAMILY

CHAPTER OVERVIEW

The birth of a child reshapes the family as a whole and necessitates major adjustments in the roles, tasks, and responsibilities of each family member. The nurse can help the family make a healthy transition to the neonate's arrival by teaching them about parent-neonate interaction and expected neonatal characteristics and by providing emotional support. Chapter 43 prepares the nurse for these roles. It describes the components of parenting, explores parenting tasks, and discusses the effects of early parent-neonate contact and sensory capacities on parent-infant bonding. It examines parent-infant interaction and the factors that affect it. It explores optimal conditions for interaction, describes the communication cues that shape the developing parent-child relationship, and examines the adaptation of each family member to childbirth. Then the chapter discusses nursing care to promote family adaptation. It describes tools used to assess maternal adaptation and the mother-infant relationship and explains how to evaluate maternal emotional status, paternal and sibling adaptation, and parental caregiving skills. The chapter concludes by presenting nursing interventions that promote parent-infant bonding, ease the transition to parenthood, and promote adaptation of all family members.

STUDENT ACTIVITIES

To test your familiarity with the information in this chapter, complete the following activities.

Clinical simulations

1. One month after delivering her daughter Abby, Janet Styler, age 25, brings Abby to the clinic for a well-baby checkup. During the history interview, the nurse observes that Ms. Styler's interaction with Abby is quite limited; she avoids close physical contact with her, never removes her from the infant carrier on her lap, and makes no meaningful eye contact with her. When Abby starts to cry, Ms. Styler merely shakes the carrier and commands her to "Hush!" in a sharp tone. Why should the nurse suspect poor maternal attachment? What are the potential consequences of poor attachment?

2. The nurse decides to refer Ms. Styler to Martha Glenn, a public health nurse, to evaluate Ms. Styler further for poor maternal attachment. Describe the advantage of a home visit in this case, and explain some steps Martha can take to help ensure the accuracy of her assessment.

3. On the day of Martha's visit, Troy Rausch—Abby's father and Ms. Styler's partner and main supportperson—is present. Why should Martha assess Mr. Rausch's adaptation during this visit? What are some specific areas that Martha should explore when assessing him?

4. Identify at least five points that Martha should include when documenting nursing care for this visit.

5. Three days after delivering her first child, Bonnie Robertson tells the nurse making a postpartal home visit that she resigned from her job shortly before her due date to devote herself full-time to raising her child. She explains that she and her husband have been married for over 4 years; both sets of grandparents live nearby, and the grandmothers take turns helping her care for her neonate, Jason. The nurse observes that Ms. Robertson is a pleasant, sensible woman who seems to take new things in stride, attending to Jason's needs with confidence and competence. Jason is a quiet, attentive neonate who responds well to Ms. Robertson's cooing and cuddling. Can the nurse conclude that the preconditions necessary for healthy parent-child attachment (as defined by Mercer) are present in this case? List the necessary preconditions.

6. Gracie Ritsick, a primiparous client age 15, delivered a daughter 6 hours ago. During a discharge planning session, the nurse on the postpartal unit asks her how she feels about being a parent. Ms. Ritsick bursts into tears. "I don't know what I'm supposed to do with the baby," she says. "My friends don't want to spend time with me any more and I'll never be able to get out to the mall now. My boyfriend's not sure he still wants to see me. My Mom says I'd better get used to taking care of the baby by myself because she doesn't come home from work until after supper." What role does Ms. Ritsick's age play in her adaptation to her new role as a parent? Explain why her reaction to motherhood is typical for a person in her age group.

7. How can Ms. Ritsick's nurse promote her psychosocial adaptation and ease her transition to parenthood?

8. One day after delivering her third child and first son, Peggy Muller asks the nurse for advice on how to handle her other children. She explains that her daughters, ages 3 and 4, seemed uncertain when she told them 5 months ago that they were going to have a baby brother or sister. How can the nurse help Ms. Muller and her husband Tom support sibling adaptation?

9. In response to the growing number of new families in the community, Memorial Hospital plans to offer a series of parenting classes to enhance parent-neonate interaction and successful adaptation to parenthood. Dixie Samuels, the nurse-educator developing the series, decides to base the classes on the essential tasks a person must accomplish to make a smooth transition to parenthood. She plans to include such topics as providing a safe environment for the neonate, learning to respond appropriately to the neonate's needs,

and helping other family members adjust to the neonate's arrival. Identify four other essential tasks of parenthood that Ms. Samuels should include to ensure a comprehensive parenting series.

Study questions

10. Explain how the parent-child relationship affects a child's psychosocial development.

11. How can the nurse promote parent-neonate interaction in the delivery room?

12. Give one example of a cognitive-affective parenting skill and one example of a cognitive-motor parenting skill. The nurse is more likely to incorporate which type of skill into parent teaching? Explain your answer.

13. Identify some assessment tools used to evaluate maternal adaptation, the mother-child relationship, and neonatal behavior.

Fill in the blank

14. Eye contact, touching, verbalizing, and exploring are examples of __________ behaviors.

15. A neonate who averts the gaze and turns away from a stimulus is indicating either __________ or __________.

16. The process by which the neonate gives cues and the parent interprets and responds to these cues is called __________.

17. __________ occurs when the parents and neonate show appropriate action and reaction to communication cues.

18. A neonate who moves in rhythm to adult speech is demonstrating the phenomenon known as __________.

True or false

19. Economic status does not affect a parent's adaptation to the neonate.
❑ True ❑ False

20. Sibling jealousy is an unhealthy reaction to the attention a neonate receives.
❑ True ❑ False

21. Acquaintance is a prerequisite to attachment and bonding.
❑ True ❑ False

22. The quality of parent-child attachment is influenced by neonatal behavior and sensory capacities.
❑ True ❑ False

23. Early contact with the neonate has little or no effect on a father's adjustment to parenthood.
❑ True ❑ False

24. Early parent-neonate contact promotes—but probably is not essential to—bonding.
❑ True ❑ False

25. A neonate's temperament affects the quality of the interaction with the parent.
❑ True ❑ False

26. All neonatal senses play a role in parent-child attachment.
❑ True ❑ False

Matching terms and definitions

27. Rubin described three phases of behavior that take place as a woman adapts to the parental role; she also identified certain maternal characteristics associated with each phase. Match the appropriate adaptation phase in the left column with each maternal characteristic in the right column. (More than one characteristic may occur during each adaptation phase.)

(1) taking in	(a) reorganizes household tasks and schedules
(2) taking hold	(b) depends less on family members
(3) letting go	(c) feels excited and is eager to talk about the childbirth experience
	(d) assimilates her new role as mother
	(e) feels overwhelmed by exhaustion
	(f) seeks positive feedback about caregiving skills
	(g) vacillates between her needs for nurturing and resuming independence
	(h) shows dependence on others

◆ CHAPTER 44 ◆

POSTPARTAL COMPLICATIONS

CHAPTER OVERVIEW

During the postpartal period, the client undergoes major physiologic and emotional changes. Nursing care during this time focuses on preventing or ensuring early detection of complications brought on by childbirth. Chapter 44 describes the physiology and etiology of common postpartal complications—including puerperal infection, postpartal hemorrhage, birth canal injuries, vascular problems, urinary tract infections, diabetes mellitus, and postpartal psychiatric disorders. It outlines nursing care for a client with each complication, focusing on assessment and intervention.

STUDENT ACTIVITIES

To test your familiarity with the information in this chapter, complete the following activities.

Clinical simulations

1. When evaluating Felice Fouillard 2 days after cesarean delivery, the nurse measures a temperature over 100.4° F on two occasions. The next morning, Ms. Fouillard has a temperature of 100.8° F, pulse rate of 102 beats/minute, respiratory rate of 24 beats/minute, and blood pressure of 110/68 mg Hg. Ms. Fouillard complains of chills and a headache. Her fundus is tender on palpation; her lochia has increased in flow and taken on a slightly foul odor. The nurse should suspect what condition as the cause of Ms. Fouillard's signs and symptoms? Explain your answer.

2. Reviewing Ms. Fouillard's antepartal and intrapartal records, the nurse notes that during pregnancy she was treated for anemia and gained only 15 lb because of her poor dietary intake. Her amniotic sac ruptured at least 36 hours before her admission to the labor and delivery area. Her labor—augmented with oxytocin to expedite delivery—lasted 18 hours. Internal fetal monitoring was used and numerous vaginal examinations were performed because of her slow labor progress. Eventually, cesarean delivery was performed because of the apparent fetal position and lack of cervical dilation. Explain why the review of Ms. Fouillard's medical records strengthens the nurse's initial suspicion about the cause of her signs and symptoms. Identify the antepartal and intrapartal risk factors on which the nurse would base this suspicion.

3. After notifying the physician of Ms. Fouillard's clinical findings, the nurse should expect the physician to order which laboratory studies?

4. The nurse should implement which measures for Ms. Fouillard?

5. Madeleine Johnson, a 41-year-old gravida 4, para 4004 client, delivered a neonate yesterday morning. Despite her anemia and obesity, she had an uneventful labor and delivery. However, on arising this morning, she complains of pain and stiffness in her right calf, directly over the site of a previous episode of phlebitis. Palpating a blood vessel in the calf where the pain is centered, the nurse finds the vessel hard, cordlike, sensitive to pressure, erythematous, and warm. Ms. Johnson also has a low-grade fever. The physician arrives to evaluate Ms. Johnson further and diagnoses superficial thrombophlebitis. Identify five factors in Ms. Johnson's history that increased her risk for this condition.

6. Which potentially life-threatening disorder might have developed had Ms. Johnson's condition gone undetected? To prevent this disorder, the nurse should implement which measures?

7. Three weeks after delivery, Janis Nathan, a breast-feeding client, visits the physician's office to seek treatment for a cracked nipple and a warm, sore, reddened area in her left breast. Her temperature measures 99.6° F. After diagnosing mastitis, the physician prescribes a full course of antibiotics and bed rest. Describe the topics the nurse should include when teaching Ms. Nathan about her treatment.

8. Rosa Ford, age 21, is admitted to the labor and delivery area with a diagnosis of abruptio placentae; to save her preterm neonate, an emergency cesarean delivery is performed. On the postpartal unit, Ms. Ford reluctantly confesses she regularly smokes crack cocaine. The nurse should expect what treatment approach for Ms. Ford during her stay in the health care facility? When documenting Ms. Ford's nursing care, the nurse should include which items?

9. Eight hours after her precipitous labor and delivery of a 9-pound son, Iris Greer, a primiparous client, calls the nurse to her room to report heavy vaginal bleeding. The nurse assesses profuse, bright red vaginal bleeding, a thready pulse of 112 beats/minute, and a blood pressure of 90/50 mm Hg. Noting that Ms. Greer appears diaphoretic and pale and cannot sit up, the nurse suspects delayed postpartal hemorrhage. However, because her fundus is firm, well contracted, and located at the midline, the nurse rules out uterine atony as a possible cause. List other possible causes of postpartal hemorrhage that the nurse should consider.

10. The physician determines that a deep cervical laceration is the cause of Ms. Greer's hemorrhage. Ms. Greer asks the nurse why this problem occurred after her quick, uneventful delivery. How should the nurse respond?

11. Two weeks postpartum, Donna Lincoln, age 28, calls the nurse in the clinic to report urinary frequency and urgency, dysuria, suprapubic pain, bloody urine, and a low-grade fever. Reviewing Ms. Lincoln's records, the nurse notes that she is a multiparous client who had a low forceps vaginal delivery; an indwelling catheter was inserted in the early postpartal period because excessive vaginal swelling had

impeded urination. The nurse should suspect what condition as the cause of Ms. Lincoln's signs and symptoms?

12. Jean-Marie LaRue, a primiparous diabetic client, plans to breast-feed her neonate. When preparing her for discharge, the nurse should include which teaching topics?

Study questions

13. List at least 10 predisposing factors for postpartal hemorrhage.

14. Briefly describe the REEDA scale and explain how the nurse uses it during postpartal assessment.

15. Which nursing measures help prevent puerperal infection?

16. List the main goals of nursing care for the postpartal client with pre-eclampsia.

17. Explain why substance abuse may go undetected until the postpartal period, when a client's neonate shows neurobehavioral abnormalities.

18. For the family of a postpartal client at risk for a major depressive episode, the nurse should provide what anticipatory guidance?

Fill in the blank

19. The hallmark of puerperal infection is ___________.

20. Once postpartal hemorrhage is diagnosed, treatment hinges on ___________.

21. For the postpartal client with pelvic relaxation, the key intervention is ___________.

22. Caring for the postpartal diabetic client can be challenging because her blood glucose levels may ___________.

23. A rectovaginal fistula is an opening between the ___________ and the ___________.

◆ CHAPTER 45 ◆

MATERNAL CARE AT HOME

CHAPTER OVERVIEW

As early discharge for postpartal clients and their neonates becomes increasingly common, the need for postpartal follow-up nursing care grows. Chapter 45 prepares the nurse to provide care for the postpartal client at home. It discusses the role of home nursing care in promoting the client's full recovery and helping her and other family members adapt to their new roles. It delineates the potential benefits of home care, including a more relaxed caregiving atmosphere, enhanced mutual trust, and more relevant care. After presenting strategies that improve the outcome of home nursing care, the chapter describes the history and physical data the nurse should collect to assess the client's postpartal recovery. It emphasizes evaluation of the client's psychosocial status and tells how to assess the safety, adequacy, and psychosocial environment of the home. The chapter examines the role of a home nursing care contract, then focuses on nursing measures that promote postpartal recovery, enhance client and family adaptation to new roles, and bolster parenting skills.

STUDENT ACTIVITIES

To test your familiarity with the information in this chapter, complete the following activities.

Clinical simulations

1. Ivy Brown, age 16, is discharged on her second postpartal day with her newborn daughter after receiving a referral for home nursing care. She lives with her boyfriend Leo Michelson, age 18, in a one-bedroom, fifth-floor tenement apartment in the inner city of a large urban area. Briefly identify the factors the nurse should assess when evaluating Ms. Brown's home.

2. When assessing Ms. Brown's psychosocial status, the nurse asks her about her daily activities, interaction with the neonate, social activities, and support systems. To complete the psychosocial assessment, the nurse should explore which other areas?

3. Ms. Brown and Mr. Michelson have no close relatives nearby and know little about parenting or caring for a neonate. Briefly discuss how the home care nurse can enhance their parenting and caregiving skills.

4. Six weeks after delivering her first child, Ginger Edelson tearfully tells the home care nurse that she feels overwhelmed by the responsibilities of motherhood, feels guilty for not interacting more with her daughter, and fears she is not a good mother. How can the nurse determine whether Ms. Edelson is experiencing "maternity blues"—a common postpartal condition—or a more serious mood alteration? The nurse should suspect which condition in Ms. Edelson's case?

Multiple choice

5. For the nurse planning a postpartal home visit, which of the following is *not* an appropriate strategy? Explain your answer.
(a) Review the client's discharge plan carefully in advance.
(b) Recognize and respect the family's beliefs, customs, and routines to build rapport and trust.
(c) During the initial visit, clarify the purpose of the visit and the services the nurse can provide to put the client at ease.
(d) Plan a spontaneous visit to allow a more accurate assessment of the family's ability to cope with the neonate.

6. Which of the following statements does *not* apply to nursing care in the home? Explain your answer.
(a) It enhances family-centered care by allowing a broader perspective for understanding the family.
(b) It is less likely to arouse feelings of invasion of privacy.
(c) It promotes mutual trust between the nurse and the client because most clients are more relaxed in their own surroundings.
(d) It gives the client more control over schedules and daily routines, allowing for the family's normal activities and requirements.

Study questions

7. List the basic elements of a complete postpartal home nursing assessment.

8. When formulating a home care plan, the nurse should incorporate which major nursing goals?

9. Before the first home visit, the nurse should note which elements of the client's immediate past pregnancy and delivery?

True or false

10. The nurse should establish definite goals for postpartal home care before each visit.
❑ True ❑ False

11. For the client who wants a less active role in her care, a home nursing care contract is essential.
❑ True ❑ False

12. Once a home nursing care contract is formalized in writing, it can be changed.
❑ True ❑ False

13. Developing a friendship with the client is an appropriate goal for the nurse providing home care.
❑ True ❑ False

14. The nurse should not recommend spontaneity as a key to resuming a satisfying sexual relationship for the postpartal couple.
❑ True ❑ False

15. The nurse providing home care should not change goals at the last minute, even if the client has a sudden crisis.
❑ True ❑ False

Matching terms and definitions

16. As the postpartal client adapts to her new role and responsibilities, certain concerns may arise. Match each client concern in the left column with the appropriate nursing intervention in the right column. (More than one intervention may address a particular client concern.)

(1) overwhelming nature of neonatal care	(a) Review the events of childbirth to help the client accept, understand, and integrate the experience.
(2) meaning of motherhood	(b) Mobilize the client's support systems.
(3) self-concept	(c) Encourage the client and her partner to communicate openly.
(4) relationship with her partner	(d) Encourage the client to express her anger.
	(e) Reinforce the strengths of the couple's relationship.
	(f) Refer the client to a support group.
	(g) Encourage the client to find time for herself.
	(h) Explore the division of household labor and suggest any necessary changes.
	(i) Help the client make social contacts so that she can share her concerns with other mothers.

ANSWERS FOR CHAPTER 1 ◆ FAMILY NURSING CARE: HISTORY AND TRENDS

Page numbers in parentheses refer to textbook pages.

Multiple choice

1. (a) (page 6)
2. (b) (page 13)

Study questions

3. *Affective function.* The family provides affection and understanding, which meet family members' psychosocial needs
Socialization and social placement function. The family provides children's primary orientation to society and confers status on members based on their family roles.
Reproductive function. By conceiving and raising children, the family ensures its continuity and that of the species.
Economic function. The family provides financial resources and allocations to its members
Health function. The family supplies physical necessities, such as food, shelter, and health care. (page 5)

4. Health care became focused on disease rather than on natural occurrences, such as childbirth. Scientific advances helped reduce deaths from communicable disease. Public health nursing also helped reduce deaths by providing home nursing care, which was vital to families who no longer could meet their health care needs by themselves. Hospitals became institutions for specialized health care delivery. Health care began to focus on expert skills, and such interventions as aseptic technique and isolation wards became popular. As health care grew increasingly institutionalized, it became acommodity for purchase. (page 8)

5. Nightingale's concepts include the nurse, patient, environment, and health. They serve as the basis of the nursing process used today. (page 8)

6. The Goldmark Report, issued in 1923, enhanced the status of nursing by calling for revision of nurse training and for emphasis on nursing education. By 1933, nursing had earned its place in higher education when the Association of Collegiate Schools of Nursing was formed and became a member of the American Council on Education. (page 9)

7. The four social trends are decreased family size,an increased number of working women, an increased number of two-career families, and more active participation in health care by women. (page 9)

8. Important issues for working mothers include maternity leave, child care, stress, and the effects of their careers on their children. (page10)

9. These two social trends are women's changing roles and the rise of consumerism. (page 11)

10. These cost-containment measures include prospective payment, alternative delivery systems, home health care, direct reimbursement, public health care, regionalization of health care, and strategies for reducing malpractice suits. (page 13)

11. Canada's lower infant mortality rate results primarily from its National Health Program, a government-mandated program that ensures universal access to health care. (page 13)

12. The drawbacks are long waits for elective surgery and treatments, and limited expensive technologies—costly machinery may not be duplicated within certain areas. (page 13)

13. The nurse can serve as advocate by getting other members of the health care team to accept the client's wishes, as long as they are reasonable.

The nurse can serve as educator by teaching clients about contraceptive choices, for example.

The nurse can act as a change agent by serving on a quality assurance board or protocol committee to make changes that promote safe, satisfying childbirth.

The nurse can serve as a nurse-researcher by analyzing current childbirth practices. (pages 16 and 17)

14. By studying women's experiences and perceptions of experiences within their environments, nurse-researchers can help substantiate women's concerns; and by providing a scientific knowledge base for maternal, neonatal, and women's health nursing care, they can help the nursing profession bring about necessary changes. (page 17)

15. A certified nurse-midwife focuses on the independent management of essentially healthy clients during the antepartal, intrapartal, and postpartal periods as well as on gynecologic health care. A family nursepractitioner has a broader perspective, focusing on the entire family to provide care for healthy neonates, children, adolescents, and adults (both women and men). A neonatal nurse practitioner specializes in the clinical care and technical stabilization of neonates and provides comprehensive case management for the neonate and family. (pages 17 and 19)

Fill in the blank

16. informational (page 20)

17. personal caring; concerned behaviors (page 20)

ANSWERS FOR CHAPTER 2 • FAMILY STRUCTURE AND FUNCTION

Page numbers in parentheses refer to textbook pages.

Clinical simulations

1. The family theories used are:
   (a) structural-functional theory
   (b) interactional theory
   (c) social exchange theory
   systems theory
   (e) developmental theory (pages 26 to 29)

2. The nurse should assess Judy's and Scott's perception of her miscarriage as a crisis, their ability to use adaptive coping mechanisms, and their participation in social support systems, such as their extended family. Their perception of the miscarriage as a stressful event hinges on their belief about its potential harm and the availability of solutions.
   This couple has experienced both types of crises. The maturational crisis occurred as they got married, moved into their first apartment together, and prepared for Judy's graduation from law school; all of these events are linked to their developmental level. The miscarriage represents a situational crisis that could threaten their self-concept and disrupt their respective family roles. (page 36)

3. The nurse should anticipate that Sylvia will have to perform all of the family functions that she formerly shared with her husband, including providing financial, emotional, and psychological support to her children. Also, Sylvia most likely will receive less affection, emotional support, assistance, and communication and may experience increased stress from her mounting responsibilities and emotional demands. (pages 30 and 31)

Study questions

4. Family theory is a set of assumptions and hypotheses that provides a reference point for studying and understanding the family. (page 26)

5. The family developmental stages are:
   (a) stage 6—family with young adult children
   (b) stage 8—aging family
   (c) stage 5—family with adolescent children
   (d) stage 1—beginning family
   (e) stage 3—family with preschool children
   (f) stage 7—family with adult children
   (g) stage 2—family with infants
   (h) stage 4—family with school-age children (page 28)

6. Possible variations include nuclear dyad—married couple with no children or with children living elsewhere; middle-aged or elderly couple—married couple whose adult children have left home; kin-network—nuclear family living near extended family members and

engaging in reciprocal physical and psychological support; and second-career family—nuclear family in which the woman enters or returns to the work force. (page 30)

7. (a) intersender conflict
(b) interrole conflict
(c) person-role conflict (page 33)

8. The three types of social support are emotional support, which involves receiving reassurance, feeling emotional attachment, and being able to depend on another person; tangible support, which involves such direct help as lending money, doing chores, or caring for a sick family member; and informational support, which includes providing facts or advice and giving feedback. (page 35)

Fill in the blank

9. structural-functional (page 29)

10. interactional (page 29)

11. social exchange (page 29)

Matching terms and definitions

12. (1) c; (2) e; (3) f; (4) g; (5) b; (6) a (pages 34 and 35)

ANSWERS FOR CHAPTER 3 ◆ NURSING PROCESS AND THE CHILDBEARING FAMILY

Page numbers in parentheses refer to textbook pages.

Clinical simulations

1. The nurse should assess Wanda's:
(a) family characteristics, by asking where her other family members live, how often they contact each other, and whether any emotional barriers exist between her and other members of her family
(b) cultural and socioeconomic influences, by identifying her and her family's cultural beliefs and values, educational level, weekly family income, religious orientation, dietary habits, social network, and child-care plans for her son and her expected child
(c) family communication patterns, by evaluating the attitudes of each family member toward the impending birth, determining their knowledge level and attitudes related to health and prenatal care, and determining their way of coping with the stresses of Wanda's loss, the impending birth, her recent move, her new financial circumstances, and an unfamiliar health care system. (page 42)

2. Poor coping skills may lead to abuse. Wanda is at risk because of the recent death of her husband (a major support person), the stress of pregnancy, and the stresses involved in moving to an unfamiliar country, which may increase her anxiety and frustration toward the demands of her expected child and 3-year-old son. (page 44)

3. To avoid an ethnocentric approach (which assumes that one's own behavior patterns or beliefs are the best or most appropriate), the nurse should keep in mind that Wanda's cultural and ethnic background and customs may affect her beliefs regarding health and illness. Also, do not assume that her health beliefs and practices are based on the biomedical model, which emphasizes technology. For example, Wanda may be more comfortable with traditional Filipino treatments. (pages 42 and 43)

4. Possible nursing diagnoses include:
   - fear related to lack of adequate financial support resulting from her husband's death and her recent move
   - potential altered parenting related to maladaptive coping responses caused by her husband's death
   - impaired social interaction related to isolation caused by recent immigration and lack of an established social network. (page 48)

Study questions

5. The nurse should assess cultural, ethnic, religious, socioeconomic, and psychological factors influencing the client and her family as well as the family's coping patterns. (page 42)

6. The three steps of planning are setting and prioritizing goals, formulating nursing interventions, and developing a care plan. (page 48)

7. Involving the client helps ensure appropriate and realistic planning, encourages client commitment, gives her a sense of control, and may improve compliance. (page 48)

8. Implementation begins as soon as the care plan is complete and ends when the established goals have been achieved. (pages 49 and 50)

9. An effective goal statement is measurable, realistic, and completely understood by the client and her family. (page 48)

10. A complete nursing diagnosis contains a problem, its etiology, and signs and symptoms. (page 48)

11. The four types of skills needed are cognitive, affective, psychomotor, and organizational. (page 50)

12. Documentation provides communication among members of the health care team, serves as a discharge planning and quality assurance tool, and establishes a legal record of the care provided. (page 52)

13. In all cases, the nurse must use sound professional judgment and document all care provided to help ensure appropriate communication of information and provision of quality care. (page 52)

Fill in the blank

14. subjective; objective (pages 39 and 40)

15. maintaining eye contact (page 41)

16. evaluation; implementation (pages 51 and 52)

17. nursing diagnosis (page 45)

Matching terms and definitions

18. (1) e (page 49); (2) d (page 51); (3) a (page 48); (4) b (page 45); (5) c (page 39)

Proper sequence:
Step 1: assessment
Step 2: diagnosis
Step 3: planning
Step 4: implementation
Step 5: evaluation (pages 39 through 51)

ANSWERS FOR CHAPTER 4 ◆ NURSE-CLIENT INTERACTION

Page numbers in parentheses refer to textbook pages.

Clinical simulations

1. If Sally's medical records are accessible, Francine should evaluate them for completeness (including history and laboratory findings), then identify any previous, current, or potential health or nursing problems to be addressed. Francine also should evaluate Sally's cultural background and communication skills. Because this visit will be conducted in the home, she may need to modify the usual procedure; for example, she will not need to prepare the environment for the meeting. (pages 55 and 56)

2. After making introductions and ensuring Sally's comfort, Francine should begin with an orientation, telling Sally what will be expected of her, outlining the nurse's role in her care, and explaining any unfamiliar procedures. Then Francine should begin to assess Sally's health care needs and formulate goals to meet these needs. Finally, Francine should schedule another visit, if necessary, for a time that is convenient for Sally. (pages 56 and 57)

3. During this phase, Francine should implement the goals set in the initiation phase; initiate teaching sessions; identify any additional goals that may be necessary; provide support for goals achieved or assistance in overcoming obstacles to the goals; and revise unmet goals to provide Sally with a greater sense of accomplishment and encouragement, if necessary. (page 57)

4. Francine should encourage Sally to discuss such feelings periodically. If she also feels sad about the completion of the interaction, she should consider sharing her feelings with Sally, if this seems appropriate. (page 58)

5. (d). Statements (a) and (c) reflect personal biases or judgments. Statement (b) is a "why" question, which the client may be unable to answer, especially at this early stage in the nurse-client relationship. (page 59)

6. Apparently, the nurse has moved into Pearl's personal space before she is ready to allow this, causing discomfort and adversely affecting the nurse-client interaction. To reduce her discomfort, move the chair further away and refrain from touching her. (pages 59 and 60)

7. The nurse should keep in mind that adolescents typically do not use information until the need for it becomes critical. They may require reteaching and reinforcement. Also, they have limited life experiences and knowledge upon which to draw as a guide for future actions. (page 61)

8. (c). Bettina's ability to listen, concentrate, and learn will be compromised until her discomfort has been reduced and she becomes more relaxed. (page 60)

9. The nurse can motivate Lynne to take charge of improving her nutritional status by teaching her about the importance of active, assertive participation in her prenatal care. Determine what she needs to know to care for herself and her fetus during pregnancy, then identify ways to improve her diet while helping her to establish goals. (page 64)

Study questions

10. The client cannot exchange ideas with anyone but the nurse, thereby forfeiting the opportunity to share experiences with others in similar situations. (page 62)

11. In successful team teaching, team members communicate with each other, respect each other as people and as professionals, use each other as resources, preserve the group's cohesion by resolving conflicts away from clients, recognize personal limits, give equally of their time and effort to promote the group's success, and establish and work toward a common goal. (page 63)

12. The *converger* learns best when presented with abstract concepts and active experimentation; she is the easiest client to teach. The *diverger* creates ideas and learns best when sharing and learning from the experiences of others; she can apply abstract concepts only with constant stimulation and learns best in group discussions. The *assimilator* prefers abstract ideas and assembling bits and pieces of information into one idea; she may need supplemental information to drive the message home and may benefit from combined teaching media. The *accommodator* learns best from personal experience and solving problems through trial and error; because she may learn best through hands-on demonstrations, she is the most difficult client to teach. (pages 61 and 62)

Fill in the blank

13. has learned (page 64)

14. therapeutic empathy (page 64)

Matching terms and definitions

15. (1) c; (2) f; (3) j; (4) d; (5) a; (6) h; (7) e; (8) g; (9) b; (10) i (page 56)

ANSWERS FOR CHAPTER 5 ◆ ETHICAL AND LEGAL CONCERNS IN FAMILY CARE

Page numbers in parentheses refer to textbook pages.

Clinical simulations

1. When confronting two equally desirable or undesirable choices, the nurse must identify the conflict,determine the underlying facts, consider possible options and their consequences, then use the following ethical principles to decide on a course of action:
   Respect for the individual. The nurse must respect a client's right to self-determination and autonomy,privacy, treatment refusal, truthfulness, and confidentiality.
   Beneficence. The nurse must avoid harming anyone and must try to prevent or remove harm and promote or do good.
   Justice. The nurse must be fair and equitable in allocating services and resources to a client. (page 68)

2. A nurse has no independent legal obligation to verify the adequacy of informed consent. However, because Mrs. Younger has demonstrated confusion or incomplete understanding, the nurse should notify the physician of Mrs. Younger's apparent confusion and ask the physician to review the procedure with her again. (page 73)

Study questions

3. A nurse practice act defines nursing in general terms, sets qualifications for licensure and grounds for discipline, and defines the powers of the board of nursing. (page 68)

4. The model proposed by Bunting and Webb helps the nurse take a systematic approach to ethical problems. Before making a decision, the nurse considers the following questions:
   - Which health issues are involved?
   - Which ethical issues are involved?
   - What further information is necessary concerning either of the above before a judgment can be made?
   - Who will be affected by this decision?
   - What are the values and opinions of the people involved?
   - What conflicts exist between the values and ethical standards of the people involved?
   - Must a decision be made and, if so, who should make it?
   - What alternatives are available?
   - For each alternative, what are the ethical justifications?
   - For each alternative, what are the possible outcomes? (page 69)

5. To win a malpractice lawsuit against a nurse, the plaintiff must prove that a nurse-client relationship existed between the defendant and the plaintiff, that the nurse violated the applicable standard of nursing care either by omission or commission, that the acts committed or omitted by the nurse were causally related to the outcome, and that damages resulted. (page 71)

6. Student nurses are subject to a charge of negligence because they are required to meet the same standard of care as graduate nurses. (page 71)

7. The principle known as respondeat superior holds the employer as well as the nurse legally responsible for nursing negligence. Under this principle, many cases involving a nurse's care do not name the nurse as a defendant. Instead, the employing health care facility defends the action of an accused nurse. Even when the nurse is a named defendant, the employer's professional liability insurance company customarily defends the claim. (page 71)

8. Mr. and Mrs. Martinez should receive a description of the procedure; its alternatives, risks,and failure rate; and the probable permanence of sterilization. (page 73)

9. The three main goals of risk management are to reduce the number of injuries for clients, visitors, and employees; to ensure sufficient documentation of client care for defending any malpractice claim; and to protect the health care professional and health care facility against financial loss by ensuring adequate professional and general liability insurance. (pages 71 and 72)

True or false

10. True (page 70)

11. False (page 69)

12. True (page 70)

13. False (page 70)

14. False (page 72)

15. False (pages 70 and 71)

16. True (page 77)

17. False (page 72)

Fill in the blank

18. reason morally (pages 67 and 68)

19. respect for the individual (page 68)

20. professional duty; possible outcomes of the actions taken (page 67)

21. nurse practice act (page 68)

Matching terms and definitions

22. (1) d; (2) c; (3) f ;(4) g; (5) b; (6) a; (7) e (page 68)

ANSWERS FOR CHAPTER 6 • REPRODUCTIVE ANATOMY AND PHYSIOLOGY

Page numbers in parentheses refer to textbook pages.

Study questions

1. The four types are gynecoid, android, anthropoid, and platypelloid.

2. In the first stage, spermatogonia (primary germinal epithelial cells) grow and develop into primary spermatocytes containing 46 chromosomes, consisting of 44 autosomes and 2 sex chromosomes (X and Y). In the second stage, primary spermatocytes divide to form secondary spermatocytes, which contain half the number of autosomes (22); one spermatocyte contains an X chromosome, the other a Y chromosome. In the third stage, secondary spermatocytes divide to form spermatids. In the fourth stage, spermatids undergo several structural changes to become mature spermatozoa. (page 107)

3. (a) ovaries (pages 93 and 94)
   (b) vagina (page 85)
   (c) prepuce (page 84)
   (d) uterus (page 88)
   (e) perineum (page 85)
   (f) fallopian tubes (page 91)
   (g) clitoris (page 85)
   (h) Bartholin's glands (page 85)

4. (a) The uterosacral ligaments maintain traction on the cervix to help secure the uterus in its normal position.
   (b) The cardinal ligaments provide primary support for the uterus, attaching it to the vagina.
   (c) The ovarian ligaments provide ancillary support for the ovaries by attaching them to the uterus.
   (d) The round ligaments help hold the uterus in position. During pregnancy, they stretch and hypertrophy; during labor, they pull the uterus forward and downward, guiding the fetus into the cervix.
   (e) The broad ligament supports the uterus and keeps it centered in the pelvic cavity. (page 92)

5. The functions of the perineal muscles are to protect the pelvic viscera; to perform the sphincter action of the urethra, vagina, and rectum; and to contract during orgasm. (page 96)

6. The cycles are the ovarian cycle and the endometrial cycle. (page 98)

7. testosterone (pages 100 and 106)

8. anterior pituitary gland (page 101)

Fill in the blank

9. perimetrium; myometrium; endometrium (page 90)

10. transverse perineal (page 96)

11. menarche (page 98)

12. menopause (page 100)

13. climacteric (page 99)

14. mittelschmerz; spinnbarkheit (page 100)

15. proliferative (page 100)

16. progesterone (page 100)

17. first; 5 to 7 (page 100)

18. follicle-stimulating hormone (FSH); luteinizing hormone (LH) (page 101)

19. connective tissue; muscle cells; elastic tissue (page 90

Matching terms and definitions

20. (1) a; (2) d; (3) f; (4) e; (5) c; (6) b; (7) g (pages 97 and 98)

Identification of anatomic structures

21. (a) mons pubis
(b) glans of clitoris
(c) prepuce of clitoris
(d) labia minora
(e) labia majora
(f) urinary meatus
(g) Skene's duct openings
(h) vaginal orifice
(i) vestibule
(j) Bartholin's duct openings
(k) fossa navicularis
(l) fourchette
(m) perineum
(n) anus (page 86)

22. (a) fallopian tube
(b) fimbria
(c) ovary
(d) corpus of uterus
(e) uterine isthmus
(f) fundus of uterus
(g) posterior fornix
(h) bladder
(i) cul-de-sac of Douglas
(j) symphysis pubis
(k) cervix
(l) clitoris
(m) rectum
(n) urethra
(o) vagina
(p) anus (page 87)

23. (a) urinary bladder
(b) symphysis pubis
(c) rectum
(d) seminal vesicle
(e) prostate gland
(f) vas deferens
(g) corpus spongiosum
(h) corpus cavernosum
(i) urethra
(j) anus
(k) epididymis
(l) testicle
(m) glans penis
(n) prepuce
(o) scrotum
(p) urethral meatus (page 103)

ANSWERS FOR CHAPTER 7 ◆ WOMEN'S HEALTH PROMOTION

Page numbers in parentheses refer to textbook pages.

Clinical simulations

1. Negative experiences with health care professionals may have reduced the frequency and extent of Ms. Thompson's contact with the public health system. For example, because of cultural factors, she may have poor rapport with her gynecologist; also, she may dislike the long waits, impersonal attention, and fragmented care sometimes found in public health clinics. As with many clients of lower socioeconomic status, Ms. Thompson may lack knowledge of her increased risk for breast and cervical cancer. Moreover, her cultural background may influence her beliefs about women's health care or may cause her to shy away from discussing certain issues with health care providers. Finally, Ms. Thompson may not understand the need for preventive medicine. (pages 111 and 112)

2. The nurse should be aware that not every culture perceives menopause in the same way. A client's perception of the climacteric may be influenced by her specific culturally based beliefs about women's roles and aging. The nurse should explore Ms. Thompson's cultural beliefs and attempt to dispel or modify any detrimental myths based on such beliefs. Also, emphasize the normality of menopause to help her develop a greater sense of self-worth, redefine her roles, and secure her feminine identity. (page 118)

3. The nurse should describe the basic anatomy and physiology related to the menstrual cycle, Then explain to Stacey that such factors as diet, exercise, sleep, climate changes, drug use, contraceptive use, stress, surgery, and illness may influence her menstrual periods. Inform her that her menstrual cycle may take several months to stabilize, and determine whether any misperceptions (such as those based on cultural myths) are clouding her understanding of menstruation. (page 113)

4. The nurse can explain to Stacey that spontaneous sexual activity without planning for contraception has far-reaching implications, including unwanted pregnancy and the risk of sexually transmitted diseases (STDs). Suggest that Stacey prepare for the time when she becomes sexually active by planning to use contraceptive foams and condoms because these methods are available over the counter, have few adverse effects, and help prevent STDs. (pages 113 and 114)

5. Joan and other women who choose alternative sex roles may avoid traditional health care providers for fear of discrimination; such avoidance may affect their care by limiting their health care options. Some lesbians are unwilling to divulge their sexual orientation to health care professionals for fear of invasive personal questions and such negative responses as ostracism, shock,

embarrassment, unfriendliness, pity, condescension, and fear. (page 112)

6. The nurse should ask Patty to review her and her family's health history and to bring copies of any medical records she may have. (She may need to ask her former health care facility to send records of her previous care.) Also ask her to bring a menstrual record. Let her know how long the visit customarily takes, and advise her to avoid douching for 24 hours beforehand because this may eliminate cells needed for diagnostic testing. Have her schedule her appointment between menstrual cycles. Invite her to bring a friend or family member if she wishes, assuring her that she will have private time with her health care provider. (page 118 and 119)

7. *Goals.* By the end of this visit, Mrs. Gunter will:
   - express an understanding of her risk factors for osteoporosis
   - describe health promotion behaviors that prevent osteoporosis
   - identify specific strategies for incorporating exercise into her daily routine.

   Implementation. The nurse should:
   - teach her about risk factors associated with an increased incidence of osteoporosis after menopause and relate these factors to her signs and symptoms
   - describe various health promotion behaviors that help prevent bone mass loss, such as dietary changes, vitamin and mineral supplementation, and exercise
   - discuss various ways to incorporate exercise into her daily routine.

   Evaluation. Upon evaluation, Mrs. Gunter:
   - stated her specific risk factors for osteoporosis
   - described ways in which she could alter her diet and exercise habit
   - planned to begin an exercise journal and to take a brisk walk for 20 minutes after dinner or before going to work. (page 140)
   - scheduled an osteoporosis screening examination with a bone scan. (page 140)

Study questions

8. Typical reasons include congenital anomaly, vaginal discharge, and trauma caused by sexual abuse or a foreign object in the vagina. (page 113)

9. An educational pelvic examination helps the client learn more about her reproductive anatomy by allowing her to view her external genitalia and cervix through a hand mirror. This may decrease her fears, help her relax, and teach her about her body functions and structures. During this examination, the nurse can dispel any erroneous beliefs or myths the client may have about her reproductive functioning and introduce her to a consumer-oriented philosophy of health care that supports her right to be informed and participate actively. This approach may influence her to seek regular gynecologic care. (pages 113 and 128)

10. To avoid trauma, the nurse should rotate the speculum blades 90 degrees and close them just before the ends reach the area adjacent to the urethral meatus and introitus. (page 131)

11. Any five of the following:
    - Be aware of personal attitudes about homosexuality that could prejudice care.
    - Develop interviewing techniques that acknowledge alternate lifestyles.
    - Seek information about lesbian culture and lesbian health concerns.
    - Expand the definition of *family* to include the people who are most important to the client.
    - Recognize health care facility policies that deny a lesbian's emotional needs.
    - Evaluate personal abilities to discuss lesbian health care sensitively.
    - Avoid stereotyping.
    - Recognize that confidentiality about sexual orientation may be critical to the client.
    - Learn about community resources for lesbians. (page 112)

12. The nurse should investigate personal habits, including the use of alcohol, drugs, and tobacco; sleep and rest patterns; exercise; nutrition; stress; and health care activities. (page 122)

13. These topics include cultural influences on beliefs, attitudes, and health values; sexuality patterns and concerns; family relationships and living arrangements; social support systems; and emotional health status. (pages 123 and 124)

14. Inspect the size, shape, and symmetry of the breasts in various positions; also inspect skin color and condition. Document any masses, skin lesions, rashes, darkened pigmentation, or rough, orange-peel-like skin. Observe nipple shape, which may vary from everted to inverted or flattened, and document any rashes, fissures, ulcerations, or spontaneous discharge from the nipple. Inspect the axillae for rashes, masses, lesions, discolored areas, and hair growth. Palpate the breasts with the client supine. Have her recline on a flat, firm surface; instruct her to raise her arm above her head on the side you will examine first. This position allows breast tissue to spread out evenly, making palpation easier. Using the pads of the middle three fingers, palpate the breast in a systematic pattern. Rotate the fingers gently against the chest wall, making sure to cover the entire breast and the tail of Spence. Repeat the procedure on the opposite side.

15. Abnormal breast palpation findings include masses, areas of induration, lymph node enlargement, and nipple discharge. (pages 125 to 127)

16. The nurse should instruct the client to examine her breasts regularly once a month just after menstruation, when breast tissue is less nodular and tender. (page 142)

17. Normal vaginal findings include rugae, which feel like small ridges running concentrically around the vaginal wall, and absence of nodules, tenderness, or structural abnormalities. Vaginal tone may be lax in a multigravid or menopausal client; in a nulliparous or virginal client, vaginal tone may be somewhat resistant and rigid.

The cervix should feel firm, smooth, mobile, and nontender when moved and touched. Typically, an older client has a relatively small cervix; a pregnant client has a softer cervix, which enlarges by the third trimester. Normally, the nonpregnant uterus lies midline; is firm, nontender, pear-shaped, symmetrical, and freely mobile; and lacks protruding masses or surface irregularities.

Palpation of the ovaries may be difficult because of their small size. If palpable, they should be oval, bilaterally mobile, somewhat flattened, firm, and smooth. They may be somewhat sensitive to palpation. The fallopian tubes normally are not palpable or sensitive.

The rectal examination should reveal no tenderness or masses. Stool should not show evidence of bleeding. (pages 133 to 136)

18.
- Concerns of adolescent women include continuing pediatric concerns; menarche; menstruation; contraception; STDs; detrimental life-style habits (such as smoking, alcohol, and drugs); eating disorders; and depression and self-destructive behavior. (pages 113 to 115)
- Concerns of childbearing women include contraception, infertility, stress-related disorders, and violent crimes. (page 115)
- Concerns of perimenopausal women include menopausal signs and symptoms, sexual and cultural concerns of menopause, and postmenopausal disturbances (such as osteoporosis and urinary incontinence). (pages 116 and 117)
- Concerns of elderly women include age-related problems (including such health problems as atrophic vaginitis, dyspareunia, osteoporosis, and incontinence); and loss of physical abilities, sensory and perceptual acuity, spouse, support systems, and home. (pages 117 and 118).

True or false

19. False (page 119)

20. True (page 120)

21. False (page 121)

22. False (page 121)

Matching related elements

23. (1) h; (2) g; (3) b; (4) c; (5) e; (6) i; (7) d; (8) a; (9) f (page 137)

ANSWERS FOR CHAPTER 8 • SEXUALITY CONCERNS

Page numbers in parentheses refer to textbook pages.

Clinical simulations

1. The nurse should inform Barbara that many couples experience increased sexual interest and activity during the second trimester of pregnancy. If appropriate, discuss the factors that contribute to this increase, including relief from pressure to conceive, elimination of the need for contraception, increased awareness of the woman's body, and celebration of the couple's accomplishment. Also mention that increased sexual desire and responsiveness may stem from certain physiologic changes during pregnancy, such as a progressive increase in pelvic vasocongestion. If appropriate, explain (in terms Barbara can understand) that in a pregnant woman, the excitement phase is characterized by pronounced breast tenderness, copious and rapid vaginal lubrication, labia majora engorgement, and a marked increase in labia minora size; the plateau phase is characterized by localized vaginal engorgement and a more rapid orgasmic platform (during the first two trimesters); and the resolution phase is characterized by chronic pelvic vasocongestion without tissue clearing with orgasm, which may be experienced as heightened sexual tension. (page 156)

2. The nurse-midwife can use the nursing process to enhance this couple's sexual activity as follows: During the assessment phase of the nursing process, the nurse-midwife asks Beth how she feels about resuming sexual relations because various postpartal physical and emotional factors can decrease sexual activity and desire. Physical factors include residual perineal pain, fatigue, or fear of injury to the episiotomy scar. Emotional factors include dissatisfaction with one's physical appearance and chronic fatigue from caring for an infant around the clock.

   Then the nurse-midwife collects a more thorough history to determine why Beth is reluctant to have intercourse, conducts a physical assessment to rule out pathologic causes, and performs appropriate laboratory tests to rule out anemia (which could be the cause of Beth's fatigue). Based on these clinical findings, the nurse-midwife could reassure Beth that her early postpartal feelings are normal and that she has healed completely, giving her permission to resume intercourse.

   During the planning phase of the nursing process, the nurse-midwife determines and prioritizes the couple's goals based on the nursing diagnosis of altered sexuality patterns related to normal postpartal adjustments. Goals for Beth and John might include:
   - deciding mutually on the level of sexual activity they desire.
   - using ways other than intercourse to express affection and intimacy.
   - discussing their sex lives more openly to arrive at a mutually satisfying level of sexual intimacy. The nurse-midwife then helps Beth and John formulate specific interventions to redirect some of their focus back to their marital relationship, comfortably resume sexual activities that are pleasurable for both partners, and foster open

communication. After they have had an opportunity to implement the plan of care, they should return for a follow-up visit to allow the nurse-midwife to evaluate their care. For example, they would state whether they have resumed mutually satisfying sexual activities, have used alternative modes of caring and intimacy, and have been able to discuss their sexual needs more openly. (page 156)

Multiple choice

3. (b) (pages 151 and 153)

4. (d) (page 154)

Study questions

5. In women, vasocongestion (blood vessel engorgement and increased blood flow to tissues) occurs mainly in the pelvic area and, to a lesser extent, in the breasts and other parts of the body; it prepares the vagina for penile penetration. In men, it causes penile erection or tumescence. (page 151)

6. Masters and Johnson developed labels for and explanations of male and female physiologic responses to sexual stimuli (called the four-phase response cycle) that are known and accepted widely today. These phases include the excitement, plateau, orgasmic, and resolution phases. Individuals move progressively through the four-phase response cycle. Although no sharp divisions distinguish the phases, specific body changes occur in sequence.
The American Psychiatric Association also identified four phases of the sexual response cycle: appetitive, excitement, orgasm, and resolution. These phases incorporate biological and psychological components, making them useful in categorizing sexual disorders. (pages 151 and 153)

7. Sexuality education for adolescents should focus mainly on the risks associated with early sexual activity, such as sexually transmitted diseases and unplanned pregnancy, and on making better choices about sexual activity and dating. (pages 154 and 155)

8. The nurse can advise elderly clients that good physical health is a key to maintaining a positive attitude about sexuality during older adulthood. Stress that sexual desire and activity can continue to be an integral part of life. In fact, older adults may be more responsible and considerate in interpersonal relationships than they were during earlier life stages. Emphasize strategies for coping with the stresses of aging and continued self-acceptance, because members of this group must deal with the loss of spouses, friends, or intimate partners during this period; such losses can affect sexuality. (page 155)

9. Rephrased questions must begin with such adverbs as "How," "Why," or "What" or with such prepositional phrases as "In what way" rather than "Has." Examples of rephrased questions include the following.
- How has your pregnancy (or illness, surgery, and so on) interfered with your functioning as a sexual partner?

- Many women notice that pregnancy (or illness, medical treatment, and so on) changes the way they feel about themselves. What has occurred for you?
- In what way has your ability to function sexually changed since you became pregnant (or became ill, had surgery, and so on)? (pages 157 and 158)

10. Appropriate guidelines to consider when evaluating a client's sexual behavior include the following:
    - What does the behavior mean to the client?
    - Does the behavior enrich or impoverish the sex life of the client and partner?
    - Is the behavior tolerable to society?
    - Is the behavior conducted between two consenting adults?
    - Is the behavior psychologically or physically harmful to the client or partner?
    - Does the behavior involve coercion? (page 158)

11. The four categories are sexual desire disorders, sexual arousal disorders, orgasmic disorders, and sexual pain disorders. (page 160)

12. Level 1: *Give permission.* Give the client professional permission to continue current sexual behaviors, and provide reassurance that such behaviors are normal. This allows the client to continue healthy behaviors and alleviates anxiety about normality. It also helps the client incorporate sexual behaviors into a positive, accepting sexual self-concept.
    Level 2: *Provide limited information.* By providing limited information on facts directly related to the client's concerns, the nurse can help change potentially negative thoughts and attitudes about sexuality and help prevent temporary sexual behavior alterations from becoming permanent ones.
    Level 3: *Make specific suggestions.* When the sexual problem is limited in scope, make specific behavioral suggestions that may relieve the problem. Reinforce existing positive behaviors and make simple suggestions for other positive sexual behaviors.
    Level 4: *Make referrals for intensive therapy.* When a client's problems do not respond to the first three levels of treatment and interfere with sexual expression, make referrals for intensive therapy with a sex therapist. (pages 161 and 162)

13. As a *sex educator*, the nurse dispels myths, corrects misinformation, and provides accurate and appropriate information. As a *sexual health care consultant*, the nurse helps community groups develop sex education programs. As a *sex counselor*, the nurse helps the client alter behavior to achieve goals and a more satisfying level of sexual functioning. (page 161)

Fill in the blank

14. attain an erection or maintain one throughout sexual activity (page 160)

15. dyspareunia (page 160)

16. lower third of the vagina (page 160)

17. subjective experience (page 151

Matching terms and definitions

18. (1) e; (2) a; (3) c; (4) d; (5) b; (6) f (page 151)

Values clarification

19. through **30.** No correct answers exist.

ANSWERS FOR CHAPTER 9 • FAMILY PLANNING

Page numbers in parentheses refer to textbook pages

Clinical simulations

1. Other essential components include Marilynn's menstrual history, previous contraceptive history, number of sexual partners, frequency of intercourse, involvement of partner, culture and religion, and belief system. (page 168)

2. (d). College students have a chaotic, stressful life-style and may be impulsive and spontaneous in their sexual choices. The symptothermal method requires abstinence required during the fertile period; therefore, it (and any other natural family planning method) is a poor choice for Marilynn because it would require her to plan ahead, thereby decreasing her sexual spontaneity. It also would force her to pay close attention to her monthly body changes, which must be quite regular for this method to work. (Stress can alter normal cycles.) (page 177)

3. The nurse should recommend condoms with spermicide to prevent exposure to STDs; oral contraceptives do not protect against disease transmission. Marilynn is at risk for STDs because of her history of multiple sex partners and her past history of an STD. (page 175)

4. Begin by determining Marilynn's level of understanding about birth control pills. Correct any misperceptions she has, and explain that birth control pills provide contraception by maintaining a constant elevated level of female hormones that prevents release of an egg every month. Emphasize that Marilynn must take the pill at the same time each day to keep the level of blood hormones constant, thus preventing release of the egg.

   Advise Marilynn to start the first pack of pills just as the physician prescribed, on the Sunday after her period begins. Recommend that she use a back-up method, such as condoms with spermicide, for the first cycle of pills. Explain that taking the pill at night with a snack before going to bed may prevent nausea. To help her remember to take the pill, describe how she can incorporate pill-taking into her daily routine by taking each dose at the same time she does another task, such as brushing her teeth. If she forgets to take a pill, tell her to take it as soon as she remembers; if she does not remember until the next day, she should take two pills at once. If she forgets two pills (for instance, because she goes away for the weekend but leaves the pill packet behind), advise her to take two pills—one in the morning and one in the evening—for 2 days and to use a back-up method for the rest of her cycle. If she forgets three or more pills, instruct her to throw away that packet and use condoms with spermicide until she gets her next period. She should then start her new packet the following Sunday.

   Tell Marilynn to take the pills for 21 days consecutively. If she has a 21-day packet of pills, she will not take any pills for a week. If she has a 28-day packet, the last week will consist of inactive pills; explain that she will get her period during this week. She should begin her new pack on the following Sunday.

Teach Marilynn to stay alert for such adverse effects as abdominal, leg, or chest pain; severe headaches; vision changes; dizziness; or shortness of breath. Advise her to call the physician immediately if she experiences any of these symptoms. Explain that some spotting or bleeding is common during the first two cycles of pills; however, she should contact the physician if spotting or bleeding occurs after the second cycle.

Tell Marilynn to call if she has any questions or problems. Instruct her to return at the specified time for a follow-up visit with the physician to make sure she is not experiencing any pill-related health problems. Finally, ask Marilynn if she has any questions, then ask her to repeat what you have told her about how to take the pills. (page 179)

5. (d). The intrauterine device (IUD) has been associated with pelvic inflammatory disease and subsequent infertility. It is not recommended for a nulliparous client who wants to start a family later. (page 178)

6. Natural family planning methods include the calendar (rhythm) method, basal body temperature method, cervical mucus (ovulation or Billings) method, sympto-thermal method, and coitus interruptus (withdrawal) method. (pages 176 to 178)

7. The nurse should explain to Cherise that she will be discharged the same day of the procedure, unless a complication develops. Advise her to stay alert for signs of complications, such as bright red bleeding that lasts more than 7 days. Instruct her to call the clinic immediately if she has bright red clots and to report signs of infection, such as an elevated temperature, pain, severe uterine cramping, foul-smelling vaginal discharge, nausea, or vomiting. Warn Cherise not to use tampons or douche, and explain the importance of wiping her perineum from front to back. Tell her to refrain from intercourse for 4 to 6 weeks, and inform her that her period should return in 4 to 6 weeks. (pages 187 and 188)

8. The nurse should review the advantages and disadvantages of sterilization with Susan and Ernie, after determining their reasons for choosing this contraceptive method. Assess how well they understand the procedure, and elicit their expectations of sterilization. Also find out if they are aware that vasectomy might be an appropriate alternative for them.

Before the procedure, describe to Susan what she can expect during and after surgery. Review postoperative danger signs to watch for, including elevated body temperature, fainting, bleeding, or discomfort that increases or persists more than 2 days; instruct Susan to report these signs promptly. Discuss postoperative limitations in activities, and advise Susan when to return for a follow-up visit with the physician. Explain that because tubal ligation is a permanent sterilization method, Susan may become emotionally upset afterward; encourage her to share such feelings. Advise Susan and

Ernie to talk to the physician if they have any concerns or questions. (pages 188 and 189)

Multiple choice

9. (c) (page 166)

10. (d) (pages 174 and 175)

Study questions

11. *Teacher.* The nurse teaches the client about the various contraceptive methods available, then teaches her how to use them properly.
Counselor. The nurse helps the client select a contraceptive method that best fits her life-style and needs, addressing such areas as her sexual and emotional concerns.
Advocate. The nurse supports the client's decision about contraception and defends her right to that decision, even if it conflicts with the nurse's personal beliefs.
Researcher. The nurse helps to expand nursing knowledge by participating in research studies and identifying additional areas for research. (page 168)

12. The five types are hormonal methods, mechanical barriers, chemical barriers, natural methods, and such other methods as the intrauterine device. (page 173)

13. (a) C; (b) CC, D, and CS; (c) OC; (d) CC, D, C, VS, CS, and NFP; (e) CC, D, C, VS, and CS; (f) CC, D, VS, and IUD; (g) OC; (h) OC; (i) CC, D, C, VS, and CS; (j) C and CS; (k) NFP; (l) IUD (pages 173 to 178)

14. The nurse must describe each method's advantages, disadvantages, adverse effects, effectiveness, cost, contraindications, and other considerations, such as possible alternatives. (page 179)

15. Possible reasons include preserving her own health or life, preventing the birth of a neonate with a severe genetic or congenital disorder, terminating a pregnancy caused by rape or incest, and avoiding negative social or economic consequences. (page 185)

16. Every nurse must evaluate personal beliefs and attitudes about family planning to avoid being influenced by these beliefs and attitudes during client contact. A nurse who feels unable to offer a client nonjudgmental counseling must refer her to another health care professional who will provide her with unbiased information. (pages 166 and 168)

Matching terms and definitions

17. (1) g; (2) a; (3) d; (4) l; (5) m; (6) i; (7) o; (8) k; (9) b; (10) p; (11) s; (12) q;(13) n; (14) r; (15) c; (16) h; (17) j; (18) e; (19) f (page 167)

ANSWERS FOR CHAPTER 10 • FERTILITY AND INFERTILITY

Page numbers in parentheses refer to textbook pages.

Clinical simulations

1. Linda's high-risk factors include advanced age for pregnancy, unmarried status, occupational exposure to potential teratogens, low socioeconomic status, more than 20% overweight, medical history of hypertension, obstetric history of spontaneous and elective abortions, possible genetic tendency toward mental retardation, family history of hypertension and diabetes, and smoking one or more packs of cigarettes daily. (page 197)

2. The nurse should gather more data on Linda's gynecologic history, including any sexually transmitted diseases or pelvic inflammatory disease, and find out which contraceptive method she uses. Explore her relationship with her partner. Also investigate her health promotion and protection behaviors, including health maintenance activities, nutrition, drug or alcohol use, and exercise habits. Finally, determine her reason for wanting to become pregnant. (pages 197 to 199)

3. The nurse should discuss Linda's childbearing plans with her and further investigate her reasons for wanting a child. Ideally, decisions about childbearing and parenting should be made by responsible adults who have considered how these new roles would affect their life-style and relationship. The nurse can help Linda by exploring the reasons for her decision and discussing its potential consequences. Arranging for Andy to take part in this discussion gives the nurse a chance to discuss the couple's concerns with both of them. During the discussion, listen actively and encourage open communication between Linda and Andy. (pages 199 to 201)

4. Topics include self-care activities, including life-style changes that would improve their own and their fetus's health, nutrition information, exercise, adequate rest, and contraceptive discontinuation. (pages 199 to 200)

5. Like other infertile women with a disturbance in self-concept and body image, Melissa may feel empty, defective, incomplete, less desirable, and unworthy. Stuart may have similar feelings, or he may equate infertility with a defect in his masculinity. A man's discovery that he is infertile sometimes leads to impotence. (page 202)

6. The nurse in an infertility clinic plays an active role in the therapeutic nursing management of infertile couples by teaching, answering questions, providing instructions, coordinating treatments, assisting in the performance of diagnostic tests, and administering certain prescribed treatments. The nurse also may counsel the couple about sexual dysfunctions, provide emotional support, help them explore their alternatives, and make appropriate referrals. (page 215)

7. The nurse should begin by determining how much Karen and Clive understand about GIFT, based on what the physician has told them. Before offering a step-by-step explanation, ask them if they have any questions. Then explain that the procedure takes 40 to 60 minutes, and inform them that Karen probably will be discharged the same day. Tell them that before the procedure begins, Karen will receive medication to stimulate follicle development. When her daily blood test and ultrasound evaluation indicate well-developed follicles, she will receive an injection of human chorionic gonadotropin (hCG). Inform them that ovulation is expected to occur within 36 hours after the injection and that surgery will be scheduled within 30 hours. Mention that another ultrasound evaluation will be conducted just before surgery to ensure that the ovaries have not yet released the mature oocytes.

   Explain that the physician will collect the mature oocytes through a laparoscopic procedure and send them to the laboratory, where they will be mixed with Clive's sperm. When the mixture is returned to the operating room, the physician will load it into a special instrument and pass it into the far end of the fallopian tube for deposition, allowing in vivo fertilization. Inform them that if the equipment cannot adequately enter the fallopian tube, the procedure will be stopped, and the sperm and oocyte mixture will be returned to the laboratory for in vitro fertilization at a later date. Emphasize that GIFT has a success rate of about 25%. (pages 217 and 221)

8. The nurse should state evaluation findings in terms of actions performed or outcomes achieved for each goal. In this case, an evaluation statement might read: "The couple successfully coped with the stresses of the GIFT procedure." (page 225)

Study questions

9. Possible reasons include the following:
   - More women are delaying childbearing until beyond age 30, when fertility decreases.
   - Sexually transmitted diseases, which cause tubal scarring, are more common.
   - Because society now accepts the discussion of sexual problems, many couples discuss infertility more openly and seek treatment for it. (page 201)

10. Cultural symbols or rituals associated with fertility include the following:
    - The ancient Chinese believed the sun and moon symbolized potency and fertility.
    - East Africans believed that bananas and figs were vessels for fertility spirits.
    - West Africans gave coconuts to childless women to promote fertility.
    - North Americans throw rice at weddings to ensure the couple's fertility. (page 196)

11. Infertility is the inability to conceive after 1 year of regular intercourse without contraception or the inability to carry a pregnancy to birth. (page 201)

12. Factors associated with female infertility:
- Possible causes of structural changes in the uterus include congenital abnormalities related to size and shape; obstruction of the uterine cavity by a narrowed or divided endometrial surface, polyps, a tumor, or Asherman's syndrome; and infections that cause scarring.
- Possible causes of anovulation secondary to ovarian failure or faulty hormonal stimulation include external factors, such as stress, exercise, or malnutrition; adrenal or pituitary tumors; adrenal hyperplasia; hypothyroidism or hyperthyroidism; and hyperprolactinemia.

Factors associated with male infertility:
- Possible causes of spermatogenesis include congenital abnormalities, such as Kleinfelter's syndrome, testicular agenesis or dysgenesis, cryptorchidism, or varicocele; acute or chronic illness or disease; stress; occupational hazards; increased intrascrotal temperature; use of prescription, nonprescription, or illicit drugs; nutritional problems; polyspermia; hormonal disorders; and autoimmunity.
- Possible causes of reproductive tract structure problems include congenital abnormalities, such as hypospadias, urethral stricture, and anomalies of the epididymis or vas deferens; infections that cause reproductive tract scarring and blockage; tumors; and surgery.

Factors associated with combined infertility:
- Possible causes of alteration in sexual function include misinformation about sexual practices; physiologic problems resulting in impotence, decreased libido, or ejaculatory disorders; psychological problems; and use of illicit drugs. (pages 203 and 204)

13. After the discovery of infertility, a couple with previously normal sexual functioning may develop such sexual problems as decreased frequency of intercourse, intercourse only during the woman's fertile period, orgasmic dysfunction, or decreased enjoyment. Ejaculatory failure is common in men who must perform for postcoital examinations. Infertile clients have reported feeling embarrassed because of the need to share sexual information, anxious over the need to have intercourse on schedule, and frustrated because of the disruption in their lives. (page 202)

Fill in the blank

14. in vitro fertilization

15. clomiphene citrate

16. gamete intrafallopian transfer

17. artificial insemination

18. human menopausal gonadotropin; clomiphene citrate (pages 216 to 219)

True or false

19. True (page 201)

20. False (page 201)

21. False (page 201)

22. True (page 201)

Matching terms and definitions

23. (1) c; (2) h; (3) g; (4) d; (5) f; (6) e; (7) b; (8) a; (9) j; (10) i (page 195)

ANSWERS FOR CHAPTER 11 • GENETICS AND GENETIC DISORDERS

Page numbers in parentheses refer to textbook pages.

Clinical simulations

1. Huntington's chorea exhibits an autosomal dominant inheritance pattern—one copy of the abnormal gene causes expression of the disorder, and male and female offspring are equally likely to be affected. Each of Ginger's siblings has a 50% chance of inheriting the disease. (page 236)

2. The nurse practitioner orders this test because sickle cell anemia is a serious hemolytic anemia with an autosomal recessive inheritance pattern. If both Sherrelle and Justin are heterozygous for the disorder (carrying one normal and one abnormal gene), each offspring has a 25% chance of inheriting the abnormal gene from each parent and being affected with the disorder (homozygous). (page 236)

3. The nurse's assurance is based on the fact that color blindness is an X-linked recessive disorder, involving a recessive abnormal gene on the X chromosome. Because a man passes only the Y chromosome to his male offspring, the disorder cannot be transmitted from father to son. (page 236)

4. The nurse should explain to Jennie and Ralph that penetrance and expressivity may come into play in an autosomal disorder, making it hard to trace. Penetrance refers to the extent to which a gene expresses a trait; for some reason, a dominant trait may not be expressed even when the gene is present. Analysis of genetic risk factors can be difficult in cases of reduced penetrance, such as in the McCabe family, in which Jennie lacks the trait but Terry has it. Also, expressivity—expression of a trait—may vary among family members, as shown by the discrepancy in manifestations between Terry and his grandfather. (In some cases, pleiotropy and mutation also may come into play.) (pages 234 and 235)

Study questions

5. In somatic cells, division takes place by mitosis, a process that occurs continuously in five distinct phases. Somatic cells contain 23 pairs of chromosomes (autosomes) that carry a unique genetic coding; they are called diploid cells because they contain a duplicate of each chromosome. When a somatic cell divides, the chromosomes replicate and separate into two daughter cells identical to the parent cell. (page 230)

6. Meiosis in the male produces gametes (reproductive cells) called spermatozoa. Gametes are haploid cells, containing 23 chromosomes. Mature spermatozoa result from a two-phase reduction division process that starts with a primary spermatocyte, a diploid cell containing 46 chromosomes. Through reduction division, secondary spermatocytes with 23 chromosomes form. As they differentiate, these spermatocytes develop into spermatids, which in turn mature into active, mobile spermatozoa. (pages 230 and 234)

7. Fertilization of two normal gametes (each possessing 23 chromosomes) restores the normal complement of 46 chromosomes in a special diploid cell known as a zygote. Transmission of genetic information from the mother and father occurs during this fusion and recombination of chromosomal material. The zygote develops into an embryo and eventually becomes a fetus. (page 230)

8. The letters are XY for a male and XX for a female. (page 234)

9. Genetic disorders can result from monogenic factors, chromosomal abnormalities, or interactions between genetic alterations and the environment. (page 233)

10. This inheritance pattern is called X-linked dominant. (page 236)

11. A three-generation pedigree is a diagram of a family tree showing the occurrence of one or more genetic traits in various family members. It is used to help trace and predict the occurrence of genetic disorders. A pedigree should include the significant medical history of at least three family generations; it should indicate clearly which family members are positive for a particular trait as well as their familial relationships to the client. To promote good communication with other health care professionals, consistent symbols should be used to construct the pedigree. (page 242)

12. The nurse should explain that genetic counseling involves testing, education about and presentation of alternatives specific to a particular disorder, and psychological support to help families adjust to genetic disorders. (page 248)

13. The nurse's roles can include identifying risk factors; identifying physical or developmental abnormalities; assessing the need for referrals to specialty services for genetic evaluations, genetic counseling, or prenatal diagnostic studies; facilitating referrals for additional evaluations; demonstrating sensitivity to the feelings of the client with a genetic disorder, especially regarding reproduction; serving as case manager, such as by helping the family find appropriate health services; preparing the family for the genetic counseling evaluation; correcting any misconceptions about genetic counseling and its purposes; and explaining the typical outcomes from genetic counseling. (pages 251 and 252)

Fill in the blank

14. gene (page 228)

15. chromosomes (page 229)

16. DNA (page 229)

17. mitosis; meiosis (page 230)

18. gametes (germ cells) (page 230)

19. genotype (page 229)

True or false

20. True (page 233)

21. True (page 233)

22. False (page 237)

23. True (page 233)

24. False (page 237)

25. True (page 235)

Matching terms and definitions

26. (1) d; (2) c; (3) f; (4) e; (5) a; (6) g; (7) b (pages 244 and 245)

ANSWERS FOR CHAPTER 12 ◆ INFECTIOUS DISORDERS

Page numbers in parentheses refer to textbook pages.

Clinical simulations

1. Several factors in Anne's case disrupt the normal vaginal balance, predisposing her to vaginitis. These include use of antibiotics, which decrease the vaginal flora and lactobacilli; excessive carbohydrate intake, which increases glycogen; and increased stress and poor nutrition, which reduce resistance to infection. Clinical findings also point to candidiasis. (pages 261 and 262)

2. (c) (page 261)

3. The nurse should expect the physician to order a complete blood count with differential to determine if infection is present, a serum pregnancy test to rule out ectopic pregnancy, a VDRL or rapid plasma reagin test to rule out syphilis, an enzyme-linked immunosorbent assay (ELISA) to rule out human immunodeficiency virus (HIV) infection, a urinalysis to screen for urinary tract infection, and cervical and vaginal cultures to identify the causative organism. (page 269)

4. (b) (page 261)

5. The nurse could suggest that Cyndy drink at least 10 glasses of fluid every day—especially water—to flush bacteria from the urinary tract; empty her bladder completely every 2 to 3 hours, or as soon as she feels the urge; wipe from front to back after urinating or defecating to prevent contamination with fecal material; take showers instead of baths and avoid using feminine hygiene deodorants and douches; avoid bladder irritants, such as caffeine, alcohol, tea, and carbonated beverages; eat acidic foods and avoid those containing baking soda or baking powder; clean the perineum before intercourse and urinate before and after intercourse to flush bacteria from the urethra; allow time for sufficient vaginal lubrication before intercourse or use a water-soluble lubricant; urinate immediately before going to sleep and immediately upon arising; consider changing contraceptive methods if cystitis recurs; take all the prescribed medication, even if her symptoms disappear; return for a follow-up medical visit after she has taken all the medication; and report any unusual vaginal discharge, which may indicate infection. (page 276)

6. Because of the many misconceptions about HIV and acquired immunodeficiency syndrome (AIDS), the nurse should ask Myra why she suspects she may have HIV infection. If Myra denies direct sexual contact with an infected person or direct exposure to infected body fluids, elicit her past medical, gynecologic, and sexual history, and ask questions about her life-style. Find out if she has a previous history of sexually transmitted disease (STD), blood transfusion before 1985, or I.V. drug abuse. Determine how many sexual partners she has had, and ask if any of them might have been bisexual, used

I.V. drugs, or received blood transfusions or blood products before 1985. Also ask if she has had any sexual partners with unknown drug or sexual histories that now cause her concern. (page 265)

Study questions

7. Cystitis, a bladder inflammation, is a lower urinary tract infection, whereas pyelonephritis, an acute inflammation of the ureters and kidneys, is an upper urinary tract infection. Pyelonephritis is less common but more serious than cystitis, which may precede it. (page 263)

8. Medications contraindicated for treating STDs during pregnancy and breast-feeding include acyclovir (used to treat herpes genitalis) and lindane (used to treat pediculosis pubis and scabies). (pages 259, 272 to 274)

9. A delicate balance of hormones and bacteria maintains normal vaginal conditions. Under the influence of estrogen, the vaginal epithelium is a thick, infection-free environment that promotes the growth of lactobacilli. By metabolizing glycogen, lactobacilli form lactic acid, which maintains an acidic environment (pH of 4 to 5) that discourages bacterial growth. (page 262)

10. PID commonly results from sexually transmitted organisms, such as *Neisseria gonorrhoeae, Chlamydia trachomatis, Mycoplasma,* and aerobic and anaerobic bacteria. The resulting inflammation and infection of the fallopian tubes may cause adhesions and scarring, which increase the risk of an ectopic pregnancy and may reduce fertility. (page 262)

11. These goals include recognizing signs and symptoms of infection, teaching the client about the infection, teaching the client how to prevent infection, teaching the client about medications and other treatments, stressing the importance of complying with the medication regimen and other treatments, and emphasizing the importance of follow-up visits to ensure that the infection has been controlled or eliminated. (page 266)

12. Predisposing factors for TSS include use of high-absorbency tampons during menstruation, use of a barrier contraceptive, chronic vaginal infection, and postoperative or postpartal infection. (page 262)

13. Consistent use of universal precautions— based on the assumption that all blood and body fluids potentially are infectious—helps prevent infectious disease caused by exposure to blood and body fluids of asymptomatic or undiagnosed clients. (page 266)

14. Essential areas to explore include the client's reason for seeking care, her menstrual and contraceptive history, any history of genitourinary problems, and her sexuality patterns. Also note any factors that may alter the client's immune response, such as age, nutritional status, environmental hazards, and life-style. (page 266)

15. The nurse should stay alert for unexplained weight loss, persistent fever, malaise, night sweats, swollen glands, and diarrhea. These

early signs of HIV infection progress toward specific markers of immunodeficiency. In some cases, signs and symptoms reflect opportunistic infection; for example, a client diagnosed with ***Pneumocystis carinii*** pneumonia may display shortness of breath, tachypnea, and hypoxemia. (page 265)

16. The nurse should teach the client about general measures that prevent infection. These include using conscientious hygiene, washing hands immediately after contact with the infected area; wiping from front to back after urinating or defecating; and practicing perineal hygiene by washing, rinsing, and drying the perineum every day. Then provide teaching specific to candidiasis. For example, advise her not to douche unless prescribed by her physician. Suggest that she wear cotton underpants, which help keep the perineum dry, thereby reducing the infection risk. Also advise her to avoid powders and perfumes because they can irritate the perineum. (page 274)

17. The nurse should inform the client that a negative ELISA test result usually indicates no HIV infection. However, caution her that a negative result may occur in an infected client whose body has not yet developed HIV antibodies. (Seroconversion from HIV negative to HIV positive can take 6 to 12 weeks.) Therefore, advise her to avoid high-risk activities and to schedule a second test 3 months later. If that test also is negative—and if she did not engage in high-risk activity in the period between the two tests—she is considered HIV negative.

If she has a nursing diagnosis of knowledge deficit related to infection prevention, explain how HIV is transmitted and describe infection prevention methods she should use. Advise her to explore the drug history and HIV status of prospective sexual partners. (pages 268, 269, and 274)

Fill in the blank

18. trichomoniasis (page 258)

19. herpes genitalis (page 258)

20. syphilis; 3 (page 259)

21. condylomata acuminata; condylomata lata (pages 259 and 260)

22. scabies (page 259)

23. pediculosis pubis (page 259)

True or false

24. True (page 257)

25. False (page 257)

26. True (page 265)

27. True (page 265)

28. False (page 265)

29. True (page 265)

Matching related elements

30. (1) e; (2) d; (3) b; (4) f; (5) a; (6) g; (7) c; (8) f (pages 258 and 259)

ANSWERS FOR CHAPTER 13 • GYNECOLOGIC DISORDERS

Page numbers in parentheses refer to textbook pages.

Clinical simulations

1. Mrs. Kayro has many risk factors for breast cancer. The most important is her strong family history of the disease: A client's risk doubles if her mother, sister, or daughter has had breast cancer. Other risk factors include age over 50, nulliparous status, obesity, and high dietary intake of animal fats. (page 285)

2. Typical reasons why a woman delays seeking medical evaluation after discovering a breast abnormality include ignorance about individual differences and normal breast changes, which may cause her to fear that the breast abnormality is a sign of cancer; denial of the abnormality; fear of breast surgery; fear of an altered body image and loss of self-esteem; fear of relationship changes; and reluctance to undergo invasive diagnostic tests and treatments. (page 284)

3. The nurse should inform Dianne that her symptoms reflect premenstrual syndrome (PMS), a relatively common problem. Explain that PMS is a physical and psychological problem, causing symptoms that recur in the latter half of the monthly menstrual cycle. Inform Dianne that by changing a few habits, she might be able to reduce the severity and frequency of her symptoms. For instance, advise her to limit her intake of refined sugar, red meat, alcohol, and caffeine and to limit her sodium intake for 2 weeks before her period. Encourage her to check with her physician about taking vitamin B complex, vitamin E, and magnesium supplements daily, to exercise three times a week for at least 20 minutes, and to practice stress-management techniques. (pages 295 and 302)

4. Common treatments for fibrocystic breast changes include dietary modifications, comfort measures, and hormone administration. The nurse practitioner might advise Ms. Charles to avoid caffeine and related substances. (Some studies show that reducing caffeine provides the greatest relief for women with constant, rather than cyclical, pain.) Other measures include wearing a good support bra 24 hours a day, restricting sodium intake, and using ice packs or anti-inflammatory drugs to treat breast discomfort. Daily administration of danazol, a hormonal medication, can reduce or eliminate fibrocystic breast changes. However, the drug can cause adverse reactions; also, breast symptoms tend to worsen gradually after danazol is discontinued. (pages 284, 291, and 292)

5. When teaching Alicia, the nurse should emphasize the importance of balanced nutrition and regular exercise to relieve dysmenorrhea and inform her that heat application and frequent rest periods may provide some immediate comfort. Mention that vitamin E also has been effective in relieving menstrual cramps, and advise her to learn stress-management techniques. Suggest an over-the-counter

nonsteroidal anti-inflammatory drug, such as ibuprofen. If these measures bring no relief, instruct Alicia to consult her health care practitioner to rule out undiagnosed gynecologic disease. (page 296)

6. The neoplasm in Fiona's breast has typical characteristics of fibroadenoma. Fiona's age also suggests fibroadenoma, which is the most common benign breast tumor in women under age 25. (page 284)

7. As a consumer, Mrs. Derrickson has the right to seek information about her disease and participate in her health care decisions. Seeking information about the disease helps clients with cancer gain a sense of control over it and increases their ability to cope with it. The nurse should provide information about Mrs. Derrickson's disorder, diagnosis, tests, treatments, and prognosis as her informational needs are assessed and her priorities are established. Offer thorough, easily understandable explanations to reduce her anxiety and increase her compliance. (page 310)

8. After a modified radical mastectomy, short-term nursing goals include promoting wound healing; minimizing lymphedema; preventing hemorrhage, shock, and infection; promoting comfort; alleviating pain; and promoting full range of motion in the affected arm. Long-term goals include client teaching and providing information about local community resources for the client's continued support after recovery. (pages 292 and 293)

Multiple choice

9. (c) (page 296)

10. (a) Colposcopy may cause cramping and pinching. (page 311)

11. (c) (page 285)

12. (b) (page 284)

13. (c) (page 305)

Study questions

14. Every client should perform a monthly BSE to become familiar with normal breast changes. A client who performs BSE may notice subtle, abnormal changes before they are obvious to a health care professional. Most women discover early breast lumps through BSE; in fact, women discover 95% of all breast lumps themselves. Women who are familiar with their breasts have discovered lesions smaller than 1 cm, which are difficult or impossible for a health care professional to detect. Early discovery and treatment of a cancerous lump greatly increase the chance for complete recovery. (pages 283 and 284)

15. A client's perception of a gynecologic disorder may be affected by her experiences, cultural beliefs, role expectations, and conscious and subconscious factors. (page 282)

16. Standard medical treatments for breast cancer are surgery, radiation, adjuvant hormone therapy, and adjuvant chemotherapy. (page 286)

17. The choice of breast cancer treatment depends on the type of tumor, the tumor stage and location, the client's needs, the client's age, the client's menopausal status, the client's general health, and the client's body-image concerns. (page 286)

18. Major warning signs of gynecologic cancer are a change in bowel or bladder habits, unusual bleeding or discharge, and a thickening or lump. (page 305)

Matching terms and definitions

19. (1) b; (2) k; (3) a; (4) c; (5) h; (6) i; (7) g; (8) l; (9) j; (10) e; (11) d; (12) f (page 283)

ANSWERS FOR CHAPTER 14 • VIOLENCE AGAINST WOMEN

Page numbers in parentheses refer to textbook pages.

Clinical simulations

1. The vague information Wendy provided about the cause of her injuries is one clue that she is the victim of abuse; her report of falling on the stairs is an implausible explanation. Other clues include her husband's inappropriate reaction to her injuries and his reluctance to leave her alone. Also, Wendy's passiveness, flat affect, and compliance with her husband's wishes suggest low self-esteem—a common finding among abused women. (page 325)

2. Walker's cycle of violence theory provides one possible explanation of Wendy's rationalization. This theory describes three distinct phases of family violence indicating that a woman may not leave an abusive situation because the abuse is not constant or totally random. (page 322)

3. Wendy and her husband are in phase III, in which the abuser promises to change and becomes kind and loving. Because the victim wants to believe that the abuser loves her and will not repeat the violence, she convinces herself that he will change; his loving behavior reinforces this belief. However, the cycle usually repeats after a period of quiescence, then increasing tension. (page 322)

4. During the assessment, the nurse collects data systematically. To help Juanita relax, focus initially on her physical signs and symptoms. Next, try to discover if she has experienced physical abuse; assure her that her privacy will be respected and confidentiality enforced. Then find out if she perceives her problem as abuse. Obtain information from the health history, physical examination, and diagnostic studies for later use in developing a plan of care. (page 324)

5. When planning and implementing care for Juanita, the nurse should offer support and information, help her grieve, make referrals, and provide family care. Encourage her to discuss her feelings about the abuse. Take steps to ensure her safety, and encourage her to take assertive action if she fears further injury. As appropriate and necessary, urge her to notify the police, or refer her for protective services, such as a shelter for abused women and their children. If she cannot take appropriate action on her own, contact community services to ensure that she gets advice on the best course of action for her and her family. (pages 330 to 332)

6. The nurse should ask a colleague to provide care, because a judgmental attitude may prevent appropriate recognition of Juanita's feelings and development of a therapeutic relationship with her. (page 324)

7. The nurse should suspect that Gina is suffering rape-trauma syndrome. In this syndrome, the client passes through three phases or

their variations. In the *acute* phase, which immediately follows the rape and may last several days to weeks, the client may experience disorganization and a wide range of emotions. Her emotional style may be expressed or controlled, and she may have physical disturbances and psychological effects. In the *outward* adjustment phase, the client may seem adjusted but is using denial and suppression to cope with the rape and regain control of her life. During this phase, she may take such actions as moving and installing new locks; these actions force the rape trauma deeper into her subconscious. During the *reorganization* phase, the denial and suppression of the outward adjustment phase no longer sustain the client. She may feel anxious and depressed, develop phobias that prompt her to change her life style, and experience menstrual or gynecologic disorders, sexual dysfunction, and sleep disorders. (page 323)

8. (a) I. The nurse should help June notify the police.
(b) A
(c) A
(d) I. The nurse must act only as an observer and should not ask questions.
(e) A
(f) I. The nurse must document *all* information properly to ensure that no important information is omitted.
(g) I. The nurse must maintain June's confidentiality and should not discuss her case with unauthorized personnel.
(h) A
(i) A (page 327)

Study questions

9. Even though asking for a description of the rape at this point may seem cruel, this information is crucial to assessing the survivor, planning her care, and collecting evidence. For instance, the time and place of the incident may suggest which evidence to look for (such as fresh or dried semen, grass stains, or dirt). The use of a weapon during the attack could help explain the survivor's injuries. Variations in evidence, such as several hair colors or blood types, may suggest more than one assailant. The nature of the attack indicates where to obtain semen specimens and check for bruises and other signs of trauma. (pages 326 and 327)

10. Sexual assault refers to penetration of any orifice by the penis, other male appendage, or other object without consent, achieved through the use of threats, force, intimidation, or deception. Rape, in contrast, is sexual intercourse without consent, achieved through the use of threats, force, intimidation, or deception. Technically, rape requires penile penetration of the vagina. (page 321)

11. Three other categories are description of the rape, specimens taken and where they were sent, and plans for follow-up care. (pages 334 and 335)

True or false

12. False (page 323)

13. False (page 321)

14. True (page 323)

15. False (page 326)

16. True (page 323)

Values clarification

17. through **25.** No correct answers exist.

Page numbers in parentheses refer to textbook pages.

Clinical simulations

1. The nurse should consider the following factors: individual food preferences, cultural preferences and traditions, social association, family demographics, product advertising and promotion, established eating patterns, allotted food preparation time, number of meals eaten at home, and availability of prepared foods. (page 338)

2. Sandra's upset probably stems from feelings of rejection, isolation, and low self-esteem, which result from discrimination against obese people. (page 341)

3. The nurse should suspect that Sandra has hyperplastic obesity because she has been obese throughout childhood and adolescence. This type of obesity is characterized by an increased number of fat cells. In contrast, hypertrophic obesity refers to an increase in the size of fat cells. Hyperplastic obesity makes significant weight loss difficult. When considering whether to diet, a client such as Sandra must weigh the emotional stress of dieting against the likelihood of regaining lost weight. (pages 339 and 340)

4. The nurse should explain that crash diets rob the body of nutrients. The body reacts as if it were starving, slowing the basal metabolic rate by 30%. This reduction in caloric use continues after the dieter resumes normal eating patterns, typically causing her to regain all of the lost weight—and possibly more. (page 341)

5. (b). This treatment may be particularly effective if Sandra learns to recognize environmental and psychological factors that trigger excessive eating. Coupled with sound nutritional counseling and a regular exercise program, this treatment results in long-term success in 10% of cases. The other treatments are more drastic measures with no record of long-term success. (page 340)

6. The nurse should inform Lila that about 80% of people who stop smoking have physical and psychological withdrawal signs and symptoms, including tobacco craving, irritability, anxiety, poor concentration, restlessness, increased appetite, and decreased heart rate. Tell her that the effects subside gradually after about 2 weeks, but emphasize that her desire to smoke may persist for years, peaking during periods of increased stress. (page 345)

7. Chris has anorexia nervosa, a serious eating disorder most commonly affecting adolescent girls and young women. Its exact cause is unknown, but researchers believe it may stem from psychological problems related to identity and self-concept; societal pressure to be thin and cultural norms that equate slimness with beauty may contribute to the disorder. Anorexia nervosa must be treated medically because it can lead to severe health problems. The nurse

should recommend that Chris undergo immediate medical evaluation—and possibly psychiatric evaluation as well. Explain that family dynamics play an important role in treatment. (pages 340 and 341)

8. The nurse should inform Betty that smoking is associated with an increased incidence of spontaneous abortions, certain congenital anomalies, low birth weight, and increased risks of fetal mortality and morbidity, sudden infant death syndrome, childhood hyperactivity, and cancer later in life. Explain that maternal cocaine use has been linked with many serious perinatal problems, including abruptio placentae—a condition that may be fatal to the fetus, the mother, or both. Inform Betty that maternal cocaine use also may cause congenital defects (especially of the urogenital system), low birth weight, and behavioral deviations. Mention that the child of a woman who used cocaine during pregnancy has an increased risk for sudden infant death syndrome and other apnea syndromes; warn her that a neonate whose mother uses crack just before delivery may suffer a stroke. (page 346)

Study questions

9. By reducing the need to perform physical labor, technological advances have decreased physical activity levels and caloric expenditure. Current food manufacturing and packaging methods add sugar, salt, fat, and artificial additives to our foods. (page 338)

10. Current standards define obesity as a body weight of 20% or more above the norm, or ideal. The norm is the range of weights (related to height and age) associated with the lowest mortality rate. (page 339)

11. Bulimia is an eating disorder characterized by insatiable food cravings that usually result in food binges followed by depression and self-deprecation. The bulimic client consumes large quantities of food, then purges the body by self-induced vomiting, use of laxatives, or other methods. Continued bulimia may cause such medical complications as gastric dilation, parotid swelling, esophagitis, pancreatitis, and cardiac arrhythmias. (pages 340 and 341)

12. Substance abuse is a maladaptive pattern of substance use marked by continued use despite knowledge that it may cause or exacerbate impairment of social, occupational, psychological, or physical functioning. Substance dependence refers to a cluster of cognitive, behavioral, and physiologic signs and symptoms that indicate impaired control of substance use, as evidenced by tolerance and withdrawal symptoms. (page 339)

13. Through denial, the abuser rejects the notion that the abused substance is causing a problem, impeding treatment and recovery; in a former substance abuser, it may promote a relapse. Through isolation, the abuser separates herself from people, situations, information, or feelings that challenge the denial. (page 342)

14. Common long-term effects of smoking include cancers of the lung, mouth, throat, pancreas, kidney, and bladder; cardiovascular dis-

ease, including cerebrovascular accidents, myocardial infarction, and vascular disorders; and respiratory disease, including emphysema, bronchitis, asthma, and pulmonary infections. (page 345)

15. Alcoholism is a pathologic pattern of alcohol use marked by cognitive, behavioral, and physiologic signs and symptoms that indicate inability to reduce alcohol intake, continued alcohol use despite adverse consequences, tolerance, and withdrawal symptoms. (page 339)

16. *Individual health.* Although alcoholism is controllable, it is an incurable, chronic, and potentially fatal disease. Its serious medical consequences include cirrhosis, neurologic disorders, cardiac disease, and coronary artery disease. An alcoholic's life expectancy is 10 to 12 years shorter than that of a nonalcoholic. To succeed, treatment of alcoholism, like that of other addictive substances, requires detoxification (which results in withdrawal symptoms sometimes requiring medication); it warrants referral to a rehabilitation program.
U.S. economy. Alcoholism takes an enormous economic toll, accounting for at least $60 billion in losses each year.
Society. Alcohol consumption is involved in about 50% of fatal motor vehicle accidents, 33% of suicides, and 67% of homicides. (pages 343 and 345)

17. These factors are poverty, career and family demands, and aging. (page 348)

18. *Powerlessness.* Women have been socialized to be physically, emotionally, and economically powerless. As a result, they may rely on others, especially men.
Limited options. Women traditionally have been taught to avoid confrontation, seek the approval of others, and respond to situations in a passive, submissive manner.
Anger. Society teaches that anger is an improper response for women, socializing women to be gentle, soft-spoken, and passive. Women who express anger may be labeled as overemotional or hysterical, and their anger is trivialized or denied.
Confusion of internal and external processes. Women are socialized to nurture and support others and to respond to others' needs. However, doing so may blur their self-concepts and create confusion about the origin of problems. (page 348)

19. Physiologic responses to stress include elevated blood pressure; tension or migraine headaches; sleep-onset insomnia or early morning awakening; fatigue; overeating or loss of appetite; indigestion, nausea, or vomiting; constipation or diarrhea; neck, shoulder, or lower back pain; hives; increased drug and alcohol consumption; hyperventilation; irritability; depression; minor accidents; cold hands or feet; and heart palpitations. (page 349)

20. Intervention strategies include the following:
Obesity. Provide appropriate dietary guidelines for reducing unnecessary fats and calories. Suggest that the client keep a daily food log to serve as a form of behavior modification. Teach about the

benefits of exercise, and develop an individualized exercise plan. Make a referral to a support group or diet workshop.

Smoking. Explore the client's smoking habits, and develop an individualized smoking cessation or prevention program. Teach behavior modification techniques for smoking cessation. Encourage exercise and nicotine gum to halt cigarette addiction. Make a referral to a community support group.

Alcohol or drug abuse. Explore the client's substance abuse habits and goals for rehabilitation and recovery. Teach the client about prescribed drug therapies. Help the client's family identify and cope with their feelings about the client's problem. Make a referral to an alcohol or drug abuse recovery program.

Stress. Teach the client how to recognize stress. Identify stress-management techniques, such as exercise, deep breathing, and scanning for tension. Suggest self-awareness and self-esteem building techniques or support groups. Make a referral to individual or group therapy. (pages 352 to 357)

21. See *Understanding substance abuse,* text pages 343 and 344, for a complete listing of signs and symptoms.

Fill in the blank

22. three-fourths (page 348)

23. physical health (page 348)

24. loneliness; financial problems (page 348)

Matching terms and definitions

25. (1) g; (2) c; (3) h; (4) a; (5) j; (6) d, f, i; (7) b; (8) e (page 339)

Values clarification

26. No correct answers exist.

ANSWERS FOR CHAPTER 16 ◆ CONCEPTION AND FETAL DEVELOPMENT

Page numbers in parentheses refer to textbook pages.

Multiple choice

1. (d). Organ systems develop during the embryonic period. (pages 365 and 372)

2. (a). The placenta is complete at 12 weeks. (page 378)

3. (b) (page 381)

Study questions

4. Fertilization depends on seminal fluid, which protects spermatozoa from acidic vaginal secretions; a thin cervical mucus conducive to spermatozoa passage; an adequate spermatozoa count; and contact between spermatozoon and ovum. (page 366)

5. The ectoderm, mesoderm, and endoderm form specific embryonic tissues and organs. (page 373)

6. A *gamete* is a male or female reproductive cell (spermatozoon or ovum). A *zygote* is a diploid cell formed by the union of a haploid ovum and spermatozoon. A *morula* is a small mass of cells that forms after a zygote undergoes several mitotic divisions. A *blastocyst* is an embryo precursor that forms when a central cavity develops within the morula and cellular differentiation begins. An *embryo* is an organism that begins to develop from the blastocyst after approximately 3 weeks of cellular division and differentiation. (page 365)

7. The umbilical cord forms from the union of the amnion, yolk sac, and connecting stalk. This union typically takes place during week 5. (page 374)

8. The two major events of the embryonic period are cell differentiation and cell organization, which lead to formation of primitive organ systems. Especially during this period (from 4 to 8 weeks after conception), certain drugs, some viral infections, radiation, and other environmental factors can disrupt embryonic development, possibly causing congenital abnormalities. A woman may not know she is pregnant until she misses one or two menstrual periods; by that time, the fetus already may have been exposed to potential teratogens. Therefore, the nurse must counsel clients who are attempting to conceive to avoid medications, exposure to X-rays, alcohol, and recreational drugs. (page 372)

9. (a) weeks 21 to 24
   (b) weeks 8 to 12
   (c) week 20
   (d) after week 27
   (e) week 40
   (f) week 12

(g) week 20
(h) week 16
(i) weeks 12 to 16
(j) weeks 20 to 24 (pages 378 and 380)

10. *Function.* Amniotic fluid provides a buoyant, temperature-controlled environment that protects the fetus during gestation.
Production. Amniotic fluid is produced by filtration and excretion. During the first part of pregnancy, it derives mainly by filtration from maternal blood; during the latter half, when the fetal kidneys function, urine becomes a major source of amniotic fluid. Some amniotic fluid is filtered from fetal blood passing through the placenta; some diffuses directly through the skin and respiratory tract. Both filtration and excretion add to the amniotic fluid volume; these additions are counterbalanced by ingestion of amniotic fluid by the fetus.
Circulation. Amniotic fluid is absorbed from the intestines into the circulatory system. It transfers across the placenta to the mother's circulation; the mother eventually excretes it in her urine. (page 376)

11. The placenta circulates blood between the mother and fetus, allowing for exchange of oxygen, nutrients, and fetal waste products; functions as a transfer medium, permitting passage of most molecular substances between the maternal and fetal systems; and serves as an endocrine organ, producing hormones that regulate certain maternal physiologic changes of pregnancy and childbirth. (pages 381 and 386)

12. The three fetal shunts are the ductus venosus, foramen ovale, and ductus arteriosus. The ductus venosus shunts most of the oxygenated blood returning from the placenta via the umbilical vein into the inferior vena cava and the right atrium. The foramen ovale directs most of the flow from the right to the left atrium, bypassing the lungs. Blood then flows to the left ventricle and into the pulmonary artery, where it bypasses the lungs through the ductus arteriosus and is ejected into the aorta to recirculate to the maternal system. (page 388)

Fill in the blank

13. ectoderm (page 373)

14. mesoderm (page 373)

15. endoderm (page 373)

Page numbers in parentheses refer to textbook pages.

Clinical simulations

1. Amenorrhea is a presumptive sign of pregnancy, allowing an assumption of pregnancy until more concrete signs occur. It does not confirm pregnancy because it may stem from other medical conditions. (pages 391 and 394)

2. Abdominal enlargement is a probable sign of pregnancy because it strongly suggests an expanding uterus. The other signs and symptoms are presumptive signs of pregnancy. (pages 394 and 395)

3. The nurse should inform Liz that the sticky yellow substance leaking from her nipples is called colostrum. Explain that colostrum is the forerunner of breast milk; it commonly is secreted during the last trimester and results from increasing hormone levels. Mention that colostrum is higher in protein, antibodies, and minerals but lower in fat and sugar than mature breast milk. Inform Liz that colostrum will be her neonate's first food; several days after delivery, mature breast milk production will begin. (pages 396 and 397)

4. The nurse should explain that increasing estrogen levels during pregnancy cause the upper respiratory tract to become more vascular. This can lead to respiratory congestion and epistaxis as capillaries in the nose, pharynx, larynx, trachea, bronchi, and vocal cords become engorged. (page 398)

5. The nurse should suspect increasing progesterone levels as the cause of heartburn in a pregnant client. This hormone decreases gastric tone and motility, which slows the stomach's emptying time and may cause reflux of stomach contents. (page 400)

6. Renata would explain to the class that hormonal stimulation during pregnancy causes the glandular tissue of the cervix to increase in cell number and become more hyperactive, secreting a thick, tenacious mucus. This mucus thickens into a mucoid, weblike structure and eventually forms a plug. The mucus plug blocks the cervical canal, acting as a barrier against bacteria and other substances that could enter the uterus during pregnancy. (page 396)

7. Renata should inform the class that hormones, weight gain, and the growing fetus lead to musculoskeletal changes in pregnant women; such changes commonly affect gait, posture, and comfort. For example, the enlarging uterus causes the pelvis to tilt forward, shifting the center of gravity. The lumbar and dorsal curves become more pronounced as the breasts enlarge and their weight pulls the shoulders forward, producing a stoop-shouldered stance. Increasing steroidal sex hormones relax the sacroiliac, sacrococcygeal, and pelvic joints, causing marked posture and gait changes. (page 401)

8. The nurse should explain that posture and previous pregnancies affect the type and amount of uterine enlargement. Multigravid clients, who have reduced abdominal muscle tone from previous pregnancy, typically look larger than primigravid clients because the uterus assumes a more forward position. (page 396)

9. The nurse should inform Betty that striae gravidarum are common during the last trimester of pregnancy because of weight gain, the enlarging uterus, and the action of adrenocorticosteroids, which cause stretching of the underlying connective tissue of the skin. Tell her that striae develop most often in skin covering the breasts, abdomen, buttocks, and thighs, and mention that these marks typically lighten after delivery. (page 402)

10. Meralgia paresthetica is a tingling and numbness in the anterolateral portion of the thigh. This condition arises when pressure from the growing uterus causes entrapment of the lateral femoral cutaneous nerve in the area of the inguinal ligaments; it is more pronounced as pregnancy progresses and as vascular stasis occurs. (page 402)

Study questions

11. One positive sign is a fetal heartbeat, which may be detected by ultrasound as early as week 5, doppler ultrasound by week 10, fetal electrocardiography by week 12, and a standard fetoscope by week 16. Another sign is fetal movement on palpation, which may be felt as a thump or flutter through the abdomen after week 18 and may be visible after week 20. (page 395)

12. Morning sickness should be considered abnormal when accompanied by fever, pain, or weight loss. (page 401)

13. Increased blood volume supplies the hypertrophied vascular system of the enlarging uterus, provides nutrition for fetal and maternal tissues, and serves as a reserve for blood loss during labor and the postpartal period. (page 399)

14. Dilation of the kidneys and ureters and relaxation of the ureters retard the flow of urine through the ureters, resulting in hydronephrosis and hydroureter; this increases the risk of urinary tract infection. (page 399)

15. The funic souffle is the blowing sound heard as fetal blood courses through the umbilical cord. The uterine souffle is the blowing sound heard as maternal blood flows through the uterine arteries to the placenta. (pages 392 and 395)

16. Skin changes occurring during pregnancy include chloasma, irregular brownish blotches over the cheekbones and forehead; linea nigra, a dark line extending midline from the umbilicus or above to the mons veneris; striae gravidarum (stretch marks), pink or brown streaks in the skin that result from stretching of the underlying connective tissue; vascular markings, angiomas that occur mostly on the neck, chest, arms, face, and legs; palmar erythema, well-delineated pinkish areas over the palms; epulides, raised, red,

fleshy areas on the gums; and nevi, circumscribed proliferations of pigment-producing cells. (page 402)

17. Quickening refers to the first active fetal movements the pregnant client detects. These movements usually are perceived as fluttering motions in the lower abdomen at 16 to 20 weeks' gestation. Because similar fluttering motions may result from abdominal gas bubbles, quickening is considered a presumptive, rather than probable or positive, sign of pregnancy. (page 394)

Fill in the blank

18. increase (page 396)

19. antidiuretic; lactation (page 397)

20. fat (page 397)

21. mechanical (page 397)

22. sounds (page 398)

True or false

23. False (page 397)

24. True (page 398)

25. True (page 391)

26. True (page 399)

27. False (page 400)

28. True (page 401)

29. True (page 400)

Matching terms and definitions

30. (1) e; (2) a; (3) c; (4) d; (5) f; (6) b (pages 394 and 395)

Page numbers in parentheses refer to textbook pages.

Clinical simulations

1. Sources of stress for Sonia and Alan include their recent move, their overcrowded living situation, economic instability, concerns for Sonia's health, and marital strain. (page 408)

2. Like anyone facing a stressful situation, Sonia will respond consciously, through coping mechanisms, or unconsciously, through defense mechanisms. (page 408)

3. (c). Enlisting and accepting help from family members reflect coping. The other statements reflect denial (a), displacement (b), or regression (d)—all of which are defense mechanisms. (pages 408 and 409)

4. To help Sonia cope more effectively, the nurse could suggest that she enlist help from experts, family members, or friends; read books or participate in classes or support groups; use spiritual resources; exercise; keep a journal; or meditate. (page 408)

5. The nurse should explain that Peter's experience, called *couvade*, is not uncommon among expectant fathers who are greatly involved in the pregnancy. In one study, 70% of fathers reported one or more couvade symptoms. (pag e 411)

6. The nurse should inform Damita that a pregnant woman may recall her dreams with greater intensity because she is awakened more often at night by heartburn, fetal activity, or the urge to urinate. Explain that dreams tend to follow a predictable pattern during pregnancy. Many experts believe dreams reflect an individual's suppressed conflicts, fears, and anxieties that are released from the subconscious during sleep. (pages 411 and 412)

7. The nurse could ask Damita such questions as what she thinks the dream is about, what it might mean, and what it reminds her of in waking life. Inform her that misplacing a baby is a common dream theme during the second trimester of pregnancy and may reflect a woman's concern over her competence and ability as a parent. (page 412)

8. The nurse educator should expect third-trimester couples to identify such psychosocial tasks as adaptation to activity changes, preparation for parenting, partner support and nurture, acceptance of body image and sexuality changes, preparation for labor, and development of birth plans. (page 415)

9. The nurse could encourage Renee and Joe to have the boys attend a sibling preparation class; involve them in decision making about the childbirth; and prepare them for the sights, sounds, smells, and

emotions they will experience. Suggest that they use home discussions, films, and audiovisual aids, such as a birthing doll. Urge them to provide a support person for each child during labor and delivery so that the children can come and go as they please. (page 417)

Multiple choice

10. (b) (page 417)

11. (a) (page 410)

Study questions

12. The sweeping changes of childbearing, its unpredictable and uncontrollable nature, and its history as an ancient human experience make it a unique experience. (page 408)

13. The nurse must address these goals:
- Promote the self-esteem of each family member.
- Involve all family members during the pregnancy.
- Promote prenatal bonding with the fetus.
- Help the family solve conflicts related to pregnancy and childbirth.
- Support adaptive coping patterns. (pages 406 and 407)

14. To promote a client's right to self-determination, the nurse should refrain from imposing personal values, feelings, and emotional reactions on the client. This requires the nurse to identify personal attitudes and feelings about childbearing and to refrain from making assumptions about the client and her preferences. Allow the client to share her feelings freely and make informed choices without the imposition of personal biases from the staff caring for her. (page 407)

15. *The health care facility.* The nurse can suggest more family-centered policies, such as sibling and grandparent visiting hours.
The community. The nurse can expand childbirth options for expectant families by working to establish a birth center.
Society. The nurse can lobby for the health of poor mothers and neonates and for necessary changes in health care by writing to state representatives about laws that fund maternal-neonatal health care and other family services. (page 407)

16. Coping mechanisms help a person identify strengths, mobilize resources, and create solutions. (page 408)

17. Defense mechanisms are unconscious thoughts or behaviors that distort reality. They allow an individual to avoid, rather than directly cope with, an anxiety-producing problem. Distorting reality and avoiding anxiety help maintain self-esteem and a desired perception of reality. (page 408)

18. Aspects of the mother-daughter relationship that influence a woman's mother image include her mother's availability in the past and during the pregnancy; her mother's reaction to the pregnancy, her acceptance of the grandchild , and her acknowledgment of her daughter as a mother; her mother's respect for the daughter's autonomy and acceptance of her as a mature adult; her mother's willingness to reminisce about her own childbearing and child-rearing experiences. (page 413)

19. Aspects of the prospective father's life that influence his role development during this time include his relationship with his father, previous fathering experiences, the fathering styles of friends and family members, and his partner's view of his role in the pregnancy. (page 413)

20. Attachment behaviors demonstrated during the second trimester include stroking and patting the abdomen, talking to the fetus about eating while the client eats, gently reprimanding the fetus for moving too much, engaging the partner in conversations with the fetus, eating a balanced diet, and engaging in other health promotion behaviors. (page 414)

21. During the second trimester, about 80% of women describe increased sexual gratification. Physical changes include heightened sensuality, pelvic vasocongestion, and increased vaginal lubrication. However, studies also show that women become increasingly dissatisfied with their body image as pregnancy progresses. (page 414)

22. Some parents choose to have children present during birth to avoid separating the children from their mother, to prevent the children from feeling excluded, to enhance the children's bond with the neonate, to build their self- esteem, and to help them accept childbirth and sexuality as normal aspects of life. (page 417)

23. Grandparents provide a sense of family continuity for their grandchildren, sharing family traditions and religious and moral values. They pass on family history, provide older role models, and, ideally, affirm the vulnerable new parents' self-esteem. (page 418)

True or false

24. False (page 418)

25. False (page 416)

26. True (page 417)

27. False (page 417)

28. False (page 410)

29. True (page 414)

CHAPTER 19 ◆ CARE DURING THE NORMAL ANTEPARTAL PERIOD

Page numbers in parentheses refer to textbook pages.

Clinical simulations

1. (c). T represents the number of term neonates born (after 37 weeks' gestation). P stands for the number of preterm neonates born (before 37 weeks' gestation). A stands for the number of pregnancies ending in spontaneous or therapeutic abortion. L stands for the number of living children. Thus, gravida 7, para 3123 indicates that Sondra is pregnant for the seventh time, has delivered three full-term neonates and one preterm neonate, had two abortions, and has three living children. (page 425)

2. The EDD equals the first day of the last normal menstrual period, minus 3 months, plus 7 days. Thus, Sondra's EDD is October 24. (January 17 minus 3 months equals October 17; plus 7 days equals October 24.) (page 425)

3. The nurse practitioner should measure Terry's fundal height at 24 cm, reflecting 24 weeks' gestation. (page 433)

4. The nurse should reassure Nina that children's feelings and reactions to the birth of a sibling vary, and inform her that regressive and aggressive behavior are not uncommon. Encourage Nina to support and reassure Kristine rather than punish her. Mention that some children benefit from accompanying their mother on prenatal visits so that they can listen to fetal heart tones and participate in activities surrounding the pregnancy. As appropriate, provide Nina with educational materials that promote sibling adjustment. (page 437)

5. The nurse-midwife might suggest that Josie use proper body mechanics and good posture; perform exercises that promote proper body alignment; ask her partner to give her a massage and apply warmth to her back; take breaks during the day, reclining on a lounge chair or her bed to rest her back; and avoid lifting heavy objects. If Josie must lift her children, she should use her leg muscles instead of her back muscles. (page 441)

6. To relieve constipation, the nurse should recommend that Pat increase her daily fluid intake to more than eight 8-ounce glasses; eat more fruits and vegetables to increase her fiber intake; eat prunes, which serve as a natural laxative; exercise daily; allow adequate time for regular bowel movements; and use laxatives only as prescribed by the physician. (page 441)

Study questions

7. When the client cannot remember the date of her LMP or has irregular menses, the EDD can be predicted from the date of quickening (initial awareness of consistent fetal movement), uterine size and growth, and an ultrasound examination. (page 425)

8. The client should be assessed regularly throughout the antepartal period. She may schedule an examination every 4 weeks until the twenty-eighth week, every 2 weeks until the thirty-sixth week, and every week until delivery. However, the number of scheduled examinations depends on the client's overall condition. (page 424)

9. The seven major components of a health history to collect during the initial assessment are biographical data, current pregnancy concerns, previous pregnancies and outcomes, gynecologic history, medical history, family health history, and psychosocial status. (pages 424, 425, 428, and 430)

10. (a) You probably will be able to hear your baby's heartbeat in about the twelfth week of your pregnancy using a device called an ultrasonic stethoscope, or in about 20 weeks using what is called a regular fetoscope.
(b) Most likely, you will begin to feel your baby's kicks between weeks 16 and 20, depending on whether you've been pregnant before and how much weight you've gained.
(c) When you lie down you will be able to feel your expanding uterus after about 16 weeks into your pregnancy. However, your pregnancy probably will not show until between weeks 18 to 22 when you'll feel the top of your uterus just below your navel. (page 431)

11. To determine fetal status, the nurse documents the client's first report of quickening, assesses fetal position using Leopold's maneuvers, and auscultates fetal heart tones once these sounds can be heard with a Doppler device. (page 433)

12. Laboratory tests performed routinely on pregnant clients include blood type and ABO group, complete blood count, rapid plasma reagent (RPR) test, sickle cell test (if indicated), rubella test, urinalysis, Papanicolaou (Pap) test, and cultures for sexually transmitted diseases. (page 436)

13. To enhance the well-being of the pregnant client and her fetus, the nurse should teach her about rest, breast care, clothing, personal hygiene, childbirth exercises, fetal activity monitoring, childbirth and parenting issues, and sexual activity. (page 439)

14. The nurse should advise pregnant clients to report any of the following signs and symptoms immediately: fever above 101° F (33.3° C); severe headache; dizziness, blurred or double vision, or spots before the eyes; abdominal pain or cramps; epigastric pain; repeated vomiting; absent or markedly decreased fetal movements; vaginal spotting or bleeding (brown or red); rush or constant leakage of fluid from the vagina; painful urination or decreased urine output; edema of the extremities and face; and muscle cramps or convulsions. (page 437)

15. Some clinicians ask clients to use fetal movement records or a fetal activity diary to increase client awareness of fetal activity or raise their confidence that no problems exists. Such methods also make

a drop in fetal activity apparent immediately and signal the client to contact her health care practitioner. (page 445)

16. Drug use, maternal hydration, cigarette smoking, glucose levels, and time of day can affect fetal activity. Also, the client will not feel fetal movements when the fetus is asleep or the movements are too subtle. (page 445)

ANSWERS FOR CHAPTER 20 ◆ NUTRITION AND DIET COUNSELING

Page numbers in parentheses refer to textbook pages.

Clinical simulations

1. The Special Supplemental Food Program for Women, Infants and Children (WIC) can improve Angela's pregnancy outcome and enhance her family's nutritional status by increasing their food intake or adding missing nutritional elements to their diet. The WIC program provides nutrition education as well as coupons for purchasing highly nutritious foods, such as milk, cheese, eggs, iron-fortified cereals, and fruit juices. It provides assistance throughout pregnancy, lactation, and the first 5 years of childhood. (page 454)

2. The nurse educator should inform Morgan and the rest of the class that weight gain during pregnancy results from the weight of the fetus and the placenta as well as increased adipose tissue, amniotic fluid, uterine blood volume, and fat and duct proliferation in the breasts. Explain that for an adolescent, nonpregnant growth gains must be added to the expected weight gain of pregnancy and that additional adjustments are necessary if she is underweight or obese. Point out that underweight women who do not gain enough weight during pregnancy tend to bear neonates at a younger gestational age and of lower birth weight and length, increasing the risk for neonatal complications. (page 454)

3. Many factors would place Lilia at nutritional risk during another pregnancy. These include frequent past pregnancies; an abnormal reproductive history; socioeconomic factors, such as occupation and income; obesity; a vegetarian diet; and a chronic systemic disorder (hypertension). (page 464)

4. The nurse should emphasize that Georgia or any client with gestational diabetes should restrict intake of simple sugars and should spread food intake evenly throughout the day to help maintain a steadier blood glucose level. Also refer Georgia to a registered dietitian for an individualized meal plan and detailed instruction. (page 467)

5. To enhance Dawn's dietary iron intake, the nurse could advise her to eat more meat, chicken, or fish, which provide easily absorbable iron and increase iron absorption from other foods; consume foods rich in vitamin C with meals; choose iron-fortified breads and cereals; eat iron-rich vegetables, such as spinach, broccoli, asparagus, and other dark-green vegetables; cook with iron pots and pans; eat dried fruits or drink prune juice; avoid foods and beverages that decrease iron absorption, such as tea and coffee; and take an iron supplement (if prescribed) with meat or a source of vitamin C. (page 472)

6. For Roberta or any pregnant client who does not consume dairy products, the usual recommendation is 1,200 mg daily of calcium supple-

mentation, fortified with vitamin D and taken between meals. The nurse should encourage Roberta to increase her intake of calcium-rich foods, because these foods provide other essential nutrients that calcium supplements lack. Other than milk (which is available in a lactose-free form), sources of calcium that Roberta could include in her diet include sardines with bones, salmon with bones, beans, oysters, shrimp, tofu, collards, bok choy, kale, mustard greens, turnip greens, and molasses. Encourage her to consume a dairy product when taking a calcium supplement; the lactose, lactic acid, and vitamin D in diary products enhance calcium absorption. (pages 460 and 461)

7. One meal plan that meets all of the recommended dietary allowances for most nutrients without including meat was compiled by the Seventh Day Adventists Dietetic Association. It calls for four servings of soy milk or soy meat substitutes, four servings of protein-rich legumes, six servings of grains, and eight servings of fruits and vegetables. (pages 472 and 473)

8. Carmen's completed diet table should look like this:

	Protein	Dairy	Fruit/ vegetables	Bread/ cereal	Sugar/ fat	Fluid
Recommended servings	3	4	4	4	0	8 glasses
Carmen's diet	1 egg 1 bowl chicken-vegetable soup chicken rice and beans	milk on cereal 1 glass milk pudding ice cream	1 glass of juice vegetables in soup 1 plantain 1 orange	2 bowls of corn flakes 1 slice bread rice 2 pastries rice	sugar on cereal butter sugar in coffee pudding soft drink pastries cookies ice cream	1 cup coffee 1 glass juice 1 soft drink 1 cup coffee 1 glass water

Carmen's diet is deficient in fruits, vegetables, and fluids. It contains far too many calories and carbohydrates from excessive intake of rice, cereal, bread, and sweets. It also contains excessive simple sugars. The nurse should advise Carmen to increase her intake of fresh fruits, vegetables, and fluids and decrease her intake of all simple sugars. Suggest that she keep a daily diet journal so that she can determine whether she is consuming each type of food in the proper amounts. (page 469)

Multiple choice

9. (b) (page 473)

10. (a) (page 457)

Study questions

11. Degree of body fat, body weight, contraceptive method, and alcohol use can influence nutrition and pregnancy outcome. (page 451)

12. During a single-fetus pregnancy, the client should gain 3 to 5 lb during the first trimester, then gain an average of 1 lb per week during the second and third trimesters. During a twin-fetus pregnancy, the weight-gain pattern should resemble that of a single-fetus preg-

nancy until approximately 20 weeks; then, weight gain should average 1½ lb per week. (pages 454 and 455)

13. The six essential nutrients are carbohydrates, fats, proteins, water, vitamins, and minerals.

Carbohydrates are the preferred energy source and serve as the body's basic fuel. Fats provide a more concentrated source of calories than carbohydrates. Proteins, also an energy source, are essential for tissue growth and maintenance; formation of essential body compounds (such as hormones and digestive enzymes); and regulation of fluid balance, nitrogen balance, antibody formation, and nutrient transport. Water is the major component of the fetus, placenta, breasts, and blood. Vitamins are compounds needed in small amounts for normal body functioning; many serve as coenzymes in cellular reactions. Minerals are nonorganic substances necessary for normal body functioning; they help maintain acid-base and fluid balance, act as catalysts in cellular reactions, transmit nerve impulses, and contribute to body structures. (pages 455 to 457)

14. The two primary methods of evaluating nutritional intake are the dietary recall method and dietary record method.

Dietary recall method. The nurse instructs the client to write down everything she ate and drank the previous day.
Advantages:
- does not require previous instructions
- does not require the client to bring anything with her or expend time outside the visit
- shows which foods the client ate rather than those she might have chosen had she known that her food choices would be examined

Disadvantage:
- may be misleading if intake of the previous day does not reflect the client's typical eating habits

Dietary record method. The client documents her food and drink intake for 1 or more days (a 3-day record usually is sufficient).
Advantages:
- yields accurate portion measurements
- reduces the chance that consumed foods or drinks will be overlooked

Disadvantages:
- takes more of the client's time
- may cause the client to change her eating habits because she knows they are being examined (page 469)

15. The pregnant client should consume at least four servings of milk and milk products; three servings of meat (chicken, fish, meat, or legumes); four servings of fruits and vegetables; and four servings of grains (whole grains, rice, or cereals). (pages 469 and 476)

16. Factors that may influence a client's food choices include food preferences; food allergies; dietary restrictions related to disorders; and cultural, ethnic, and religious factors. (page 472)

17. Fluid needs vary according to age, weight, climate, and activity. However, a basic guideline is 1 liter of fluid for every 1,000 calories consumed. (page 457)

Page numbers in parentheses refer to textbook pages.

Clinical simulations

1. Five overall educational goals that Ina likely will develop include enabling the client or couple to make informed choices about childbearing and child rearing based on accurate, scientific, and practical information; follow an antepartal health regimen that includes appropriate nutrition, exercise, rest, health care, and psychological development; cope effectively with pregnancy, labor, and childbirth; deal positively with infant care and other demands of early parenthood; and make the transition from expectant parent to parent who is responsible for a neonate. (page 480)

2. (1) a through n; (2) c, k; (3) a, b, d, f, g, h, i, m; (4) e, f, j; (5) e, f, h, l, n (page 480)

3. The common goal of all of these topics is enabling the client or couple to make informed choices about childbearing and child rearing. To meet this goal, Ina consistently must provide accurate, scientific, and practical information. (page 480)

4. Lynne could meet her clients' teaching needs through the following educator roles:
   Childbirth educator. In this role, Lynne would teach preparation for childbirth and parenting. To prepare for this role, Lynne would attend a continuing education program and receive certification by an organization such as the International Childbirth Education Association or the American Society for Psychoprophylaxis in Obstetrics.
   Education coordinator. In this capacity, Lynne would plan and implement educational programs covering various childbearing and child rearing issues. She would have to complete continuing education programs or obtain a master's degree in nursing or a related field.
   Lactation consultant. In this role, Lynne would provide information and support to pregnant and postpartal women who wish to breastfeed. To prepare for this role, she would obtain continuing education credits and certification by the International Lactation Consultant Association.
   Montrice. In this role, Lynne would provide professional support for clients in labor. To prepare for this role, she would serve an apprenticeship with another nurse or childbirth educator who is a montrice. (page 482)

5. Joyce must assume that her students will have these learning characteristics: a perspective limited to direct personal experiences; a need for specific and concrete terms, rather than abstract information; and a tendency to present information in bits and pieces without indentifiable patterns or logical connections. (page 482)

Study questions

6. The purpose of childbirth education is to improve the health and well-being of the pregnant client, her fetus, and her family by providing information about conception, pregnancy, childbirth, and family life. Childbirth education encourages the client's and family's active participation and decision making in their care by teaching them about various aspects of childbearing and child rearing. (page 480)

7. The nurse must assess each family member's educational level, experience with childbirth education, perceived needs, and motivation to learn. Then evaluate the family's cultural background and financial, social, developmental, and psychological status. (pages 482 and 483)

8. Six components commonly incorporated into every childbirth education course include the physiologic aspects of pregnancy and childbirth, relaxation techniques, breathing techniques, posture and body mechanics, exercise, and the transition to parenthood. (page 483)

9. In patterned paced breathing, begin each contraction with a deep cleansing breath; use an internal or external focal point to help concentrate on breathing and relaxation. Take a series of three to six modified paced breaths followed by a soft exhalation, or blow, to mark the end of the pattern. Breathe in time to music or vary the pattern as desired. Remain relaxed while breathing and maintain a constant respiratory rate. Do not force any particular sound when breathing. Accentuate the exhalation every three to six breaths. Do not exhale too forcefully or breathe too rapidly, or you may hyperventilate. Report any symptoms of hyperventilation, such as dizziness and tingling in the hands, feet, or face. Finish the contraction with a deep cleansing breath. (pages 489 and 490)

10. For this exercise, the client positions herself on her hands and knees with her head and back parallel to the floor. Then she tightens her stomach muscles and tucks her buttocks under to round the lower back. She holds this position for a slow count of 5, then releases. (She should not hold her breath.) She repeats the exercise five times at first, then builds to ten repetitions. (page 495)

11. Discussing the transition to parenthood can help expectant couples assess their support systems, mobilize support, identify ways to strengthen support, and anticipate the types of support they will need when they become parents. (page 493)

12. Four tasks that prepare the expectant client for the maternal role include seeking safe passage for herself and the child, ensuring acceptance of the child by significant others, bonding with the unknown child, and learning to give of herself. (page 493)

13. Issues that can lead to role conflicts for expectant mothers include the concept of a good mother, lack of maternal role models, conflicts between career and parenting, and infant feeding methods. Issues that can lead to role conflicts for expectant fathers include

the concept of a good father as provider and protector, lack of paternal role models, fantasies about the neonate and his interactions with the neonate, and the added responsibilities of fatherhood. (pages 493 and 500)

Matching terms and definitions

14. (1) c; (2) e; (3) a; (4) d; (5) b (page 482)

15. (1) f; (2) d; (3) a; (4) e; (5) g; (6) e; (7) b (page 501)

Values clarification

16. through **25.** No correct answers exist.

ANSWERS FOR CHAPTER 22 • HIGH-RISK ANTEPARTAL CLIENTS

Page numbers in parentheses refer to textbook pages

Clinical simulations

1. Heather and other pregnant adolescents are at risk because of their physical and psychological immaturity, potential for pregnancy complications, lack of prenatal care, and lack of social and economic support systems. The risks Heather faces include pregnancy-induced hypertension (PIH), iron deficiency anemia, a sexually transmitted disease, and cephalopelvic disproportion; her neonate is at risk for prematurity and low birth weight. Also, she may drop out of school to care for her child, which eventually may affect her quality of life, job opportunities and advancements, and economic stability. (pages 507 and 508)

2. To promote a healthier outcome for Heather, the nurse can:
   - provide prenatal education about pregnancy, fetal development, birth, and infant care
   - urge her to obtain consistent prenatal care throughout the remainder of her pregnancy
   - discuss other options, such as adoption, as she requests
   - encourage her to stay in school to help her mature and increase her career opportunities
   - provide counseling to help her plan to meet her parenting responsibilities
   - suggest that she join a peer support group
   - provide her with a social service referral to obtain financial assistance
   - promote her self-esteem and assist with decision making and problem solving
   - teach her to recognize and report pregnancy complications
   - arrange for family counseling to discuss problems and maintain family unity. (page 507)

3. The nurse should explain to the DeSantos that amniocentesis is an invasive test used to detect genetic disorders and diagnose various fetal defects by chromosomal analysis of fetal cells. Inform them that a sample of amniotic fluid will be withdrawn from the amniotic sac through a special needle placed through Mary's abdomen into the uterus. Mention that test results may take 2 to 4 weeks. Advise Mary of potential complications of the procedure, such as trauma to herself, her fetus, the umbilical cord, or placenta; spontaneous abortion; and infection. However, tell her that abdominal ultrasound will be used to help prevent trauma. Encourage her to stay alert for decreased fetal movement, persistent uterine contractions, and abdominal discomfort after the procedure; instruct her to return immediately for evaluation if these occur. (pages 528, 530, and 531)

4. The nurse should expect the physician to order tests to determine the well-being of Helen's fetus, such as ultrasonography, a biophysi-

cal profile (BPP), fetal movement count, non-stress test (NST), nipple stimulation contraction stress test, or, if needed, an oxytocin contraction test. (page 513)

5. Ruby's complaints strongly suggest iron deficiency anemia. This condition is diagnosed by blood tests after a thorough history and physical examination are conducted. Laboratory tests typically include hemoglobin electrophoresis, complete blood count with differential, and folic acid and serum iron measurements. (pages 514 and 527)

6. Without treatment, Ruby may suffer fatigue and poor tissue integrity resulting in tissue damage during delivery. She may be at increased risk for antepartal or postpartal infection with impaired healing, as well as excessive postpartal bleeding. Risks to her fetus or neonate include fetal distress from hypoxia and (with severe, untreated anemia) stillbirth or a small-for-gestational-age neonate. (page 514)

7. During her pregnancy, Ruby should receive a supplement of 200 mg of elemental iron—supplied in 1 g of ferrous sulfate or 2 g of ferrous gluconate—to maintain normal hemoglobin concentration. When teaching Ruby, instruct her to report any signs of bleeding, especially vaginal bleeding. Advise her to take iron supplements in divided doses to help prevent or decrease adverse gastrointestinal effects. Urge her to take the supplements with an acidic juice (such as orange juice) to enhance its absorption and to avoid taking them with dairy products. Inform her that iron may turn her stool black and cause constipation. Recommend that she include iron-rich foods in her diet and consume more fluids, fiber, and fruits to avoid constipation. Urge her to comply with treatment. (pages 514 and 532)

8. The nurse should determine if Jill has a nursing diagnosis of ***knowledge deficit related to fetal effects of alcohol abuse***. If she does, teach her about the adverse effects of alcohol abuse on her and her fetus or neonate. For instance, inform her that her fetus is at risk for stillbirth, intrauterine growth retardation, short palpebral fissures, microcephaly, irritability, poor coordination, and fetal alcohol syndrome. Encourage her to seek treatment or join an alcohol-abuse program. (pages 522 and 534)

Multiple choice

9. (c) Increased moderate exercise, not bed rest, is recommended for pregnant diabetic clients. (page 513)

10. (d) (page 523)

Study questions

11. Common surgical procedures performed on pregnant clients include ovarian cyst removal, acute appendectomy, breast surgery, repair of an incompetent cervix, and surgery for cholecystitis. (page 523)

12. The BPP is used to predict perinatal asphyxia, assess fetal risks, and detect fetal anomalies. It assesses the following variables: fetal breathing movements, gross body movements, fetal tone, reactive

fetal heart rate (FHR), and qualitative amniotic fluid volume. (page 529)

13. In an NST, a reactive (favorable) result shows two to three FHR increases of 15 or more beats/minute, lasting for 15 seconds or more, over 20 to 30 minutes. These increases occur with fetal movement. A nonreactive (unfavorable) result occurs when the FHR does not increase by 15 or more beats/minute over the specified time. A nonreactive NST may indicate fetal hypoxia.
In a nipple stimulation contraction stress test, a negative (favorable) result indicates that no late FHR decelerations occur with contractions. With a positive (unfavorable) result, late decelerations accompany contractions, indicating possible uteroplacental insufficiency. (page 529)

14. TORCH is an acronym for toxoplasmosis, other infections (chlamydia, group B beta hemolytic streptococcus, syphilis, and varicella zoster), rubella, cytomegalovirus, and herpesvirus type 2 infections. TORCH infections can cause major congenital anomalies or death in the embryo or fetus. (page 521)

15. Accidental injury and physical abuse are primary causes of trauma in pregnant clients. (page 523)

16. Sickle cell crisis is most likely to occur during the second half of pregnancy, although it may occur at any time. (page 515)

17. Effects of diabetes mellitus depend on disease severity. When uncontrolled or associated with vascular damage, diabetes increases the risk of pregnancy complications. For example, it can cause maternal hyperglycemia leading to ketosis; unless treated, the client may become comatose and she or her fetus may die. Other maternal effects of diabetes include hydramnios, which may increase maternal discomfort later in pregnancy and cause premature rupture of the membranes and premature labor; PIH; and glycosuria, which predisposes the client to monilia vaginitis and urinary tract infections. (page 512)

18. Mortality increases in the client with active rheumatic heart disease during pregnancy as well as one with a higher functional classification of the disease. Functional class I carries only a 0.1% maternal mortality rate; class IV, a 6% mortality rate. (page 511)

19. The pregnant client with cardiac disease must be monitored regularly. Depending on her condition, she may benefit from bed rest, fluid restrictions, proper nutrition, and certain medications (such as digitalis, diuretics, antiarrhythmics, antibiotics, and anticoagulants). (pages 510 and 538)

True or false

20. False (page 509)

21. True (page 509)

22. True (page 513)

23. True (page 512)

24. False (page 511)

25. False (page 518)

26. True (page 518)

27. False (page 519)

28. True (page 521)

ANSWERS FOR CHAPTER 23 • ANTEPARTAL COMPLICATIONS

Page numbers in parentheses refer to textbook pages.

Clinical simulations

1. The two most common causes of bleeding during the first trimester are spontaneous abortion and ectopic pregnancy. The nurse should arrange for Stephanie to see the physician immediately because she may need emergency medical intervention to avoid complications. (pages 545 and 562)

2. The nurse should expect the physician to order all or a combination of the following: bed rest; sedation; decreased stress; and avoidance of sexual intercourse, douches, and cathartics.

   The nurse should reinforce the physician's management plan with Stephanie while maintaining a calm, confident, and sympathetic manner. Because even small amounts of visible blood can be frightening to the pregnant client, provide Stephanie and her family with frequent, complete information about the plan of care, its rationale, and her progress. Encourage her to maintain bed rest and decrease her stress and anxiety as much as possible. Instruct her to report such warning signs as pain and heavy bleeding to ensure prompt evaluation. Advise her to save any expelled tissue. (pages 545, 547, and 562)

3. The nurse suspects PIH because of Delores's elevated blood pressure and its time of onset, coupled with such risk factors as her age, primigravidity, multiple gestation, and past history of hypertensive vascular disease. (pages 551 and 560)

4. The nurse should evaluate Delores for proteinuria and edema, especially of the face and hands. Ask her if she has experienced headaches; dizziness; visual disturbances; irritability; swelling of the face, hands, or feet; or epigastric pain. Assess her deep tendon reflexes for hyporeflexia or hyperreflexia, and evaluate her weight gain trends and proteinuria. (page 560)

5. Nursing goals for Delores include preventing eclampsia and seizures, ensuring her survival with minimal morbidity, promoting as mature a birth as possible for her twins, and avoiding significant postpartal complications. (page 570)

6. Karline requires increased antepartal surveillance for preterm labor because seven of her history factors fall into the low-risk category for preterm labor; two or more factors in this category call for increased antepartal surveillance. Karline's low-risk factors include her age, low socioeconomic status, single marital status, height and weight, cigarette smoking, and a history suggestive of pyelonephritis. (page 559)

7. The nurse should inform Karline that in-home uterine monitoring is an intensive perinatal nursing service that allows outpatient assess-

ment of uterine activity with a lightweight monitoring system. It incorporates 24-hour nursing availability, daily transmission of recorded uterine activity, physician consultation as needed, weekly physician updates, and ongoing client teaching and reinforcement of the treatment plan. Inform Karline that she will monitor herself for 1 hour each morning and each evening and will be taught to recognize early labor signs and symptoms. She will transmit monitoring data by telephone to the nurse, who will evaluate the number of contractions. If she has more than three contractions in 1 hour, she will be instructed to force fluids immediately, empty her bladder, lie on her left side, and monitor her responses. If a second transmission of the same uterine activity follows, the physician or nurse-midwife will be notified. Inform Karline that at-home uterine monitoring is more cost-effective and less complicated than hospitalization and will allow her to participate actively in her own care. (pages 566 and 568)

8. The nurse should monitor Barbara's vital signs every 15 minutes, or as prescribed, and collect appropriate laboratory data, as ordered. (Laboratory tests might include a complete blood count with differential, blood type, Rh, crossmatch, and serum human chorionic gonadotropin). Prepare an I.V. fluid infusion with a large-bore needle to accommodate blood transfusions, if needed, and a medication port. Have oxygen at hand to prevent hypoxia related to hypovolemia, and gather emergency medications and equipment in case of shock. Prepare Barbara for surgery, as ordered, by explaining the procedure, ensuring that she has given consent, administering prescribed preoperative medication, and completing the surgical checklist. Keep her and her family informed. (page 563)

9. The nurse should gather information about Catherine's previous pregnancies, especially those that ended in abortions. Determine if Rh sensitization occurred during a previous pregnancy or if she delivered a neonate with hemolytic disease. Also find out if she received RhIg during or after a previous pregnancy, and note whether she received any blood replacement therapy. (pages 560 and 571)

Multiple choice

10. (d) (page 546)

11. (a) (page 546)

12. (c) (page 566)

Study questions

13. PROM refers to rupture of the amniotic sac before onset of labor, independent of the length of gestation. Maternal risks of PROM include maternal morbidity and mortality, mainly because of the increased chance for infection. Fetal and neonatal risks include sepsis, preterm delivery, anoxia, respiratory distress syndrome, cord prolapse, and traumatic delivery. (page 548)

14. Appendicitis, salpingitis, abortion, ovarian cysts, and urinary tract infections can mimic a ruptured ectopic pregnancy. (pages 555 and 557)

15. Causes of recurrent (habitual) abortion include genetic factors (chromosomal aberrations), anomalies of the reproductive tract (double uterus and its variants), an incompetent cervix, endocrine imbalances (such as hypothyroidism or diabetes mellitus), and systemic disorders (such as lupus erythematosus). (page 545)

16. The McDonald procedure is transvaginal cervical cerclage. In this procedure, a band of nonabsorbable ribbon is placed around the cervix beneath the mucosa to constrict the opening. The suture works much like a drawstring. The key to its success is placing the suture high enough on the cervix so that it will stay in place. The McDonald procedure typically is delayed until the client is 14 to 16 weeks pregnant to eliminate the need to remove the suture for a spontaneous first-trimester abortion. (page 565)

17. Potential consequences of untreated hyperemesis gravidarum include maternal dehydration, which ultimately decreases the circulating blood volume; confusion, coma, and hepatic and renal failure may ensue. When hyperemesis gravidarum is suspected, the nurse should check for signs of progressive dehydration and impending hypovolemia, such as weight loss, increased pulse rate, decreased blood pressure, skin turgor changes, and dry mucous membranes. (page 559)

18. Factors that may contribute to the onset of preterm labor and delivery include pneumonia, appendicitis with sepsis, other acute infections, multiple gestation, grand multiparity, teenage pregnancy, uterine anomalies, poverty, smoking, alcohol abuse, drug addiction, and psychological trauma. (page 549)

19. Adverse effects of beta-adrenergic agonists include tachycardia, hypotension, bronchial dilation, increased plasma volume, increased cardiac output, arrhythmias, myocardial ischemia, reduced urine output, restlessness, headache, nausea, and vomiting. (page 567)

20. To determine PIH, Remich and Youngkin subtracted the first calculated MAP from the highest recorded MAP; if the difference was 20 mm Hg or higher, the researchers determined that PIH was present. Monitoring and analyzing MAP changes throughout pregnancy could prove to be an effective, low-cost, and low-risk predictive test for the development of PIH. (page 560)

21. Factors that have significantly reduced the mortality rate for hemolytic disease of the newborn include amniocentesis studies, early delivery of affected fetuses, and exchange or replacement transfusions. (page 554)

True or false

22. True (page 545)

23. False (page 546)

24. True (page 549)

25. True (page 548)

26. False (page 550)

27. False (page 549)

28. True (page 558)

ANSWERS FOR CHAPTER 24 ♦ PHYSIOLOGY OF LABOR AND CHILDBIRTH

Page numbers in parentheses refer to textbook pages.

Clinical simulations

1. Premonitory signs and symptoms include lightening, increased Braxton Hicks contractions, mucus plug dislodgment, bloody show, spontaneous rupture of the membranes, weight loss, and the nesting instinct. (pages 585 and 586)

2. Melinda explains that these contractions, called Braxton Hicks contractions, typically occur throughout pregnancy. In a primiparous client, they become more noticeable during the last 6 weeks of pregnancy. Although they do not cause cervical dilation, they "ripen" the cervix, loosening its fibrous connective tissue and making it softer, thinner, shorter, and more pliable. (pages 585 and 586)

3. The nurse should inform Sharon that cervical effacement and dilation are caused by myometrial activity at the onset of labor. Mention that effacement refers to progressive shortening of the vaginal portion of the cervix and thinning of its walls as it is stretched by the fetus during labor. Tell Sharon that effacement is described as a percentage. With 100% effacement, her cervix is paper thin and continuous with the lower uterine segment.
   Explain that dilation refers to progressive enlargement of the cervix from less than 1 cm to about 10 cm to allow the fetus to pass from the uterus into the birth canal. Tell Sharon that at 5 cm dilation, her cervix has opened half way. (page 587)

4. The nurse-midwife should tell Debra and Stephen that the pelvic diameters are affected by maternal position during labor, the hormone relaxin, and the amount of fat or soft tissue surrounding the pelvis. Assuming a squatting or lateral Sim's position may help increase these diameters. The nurse-midwife should mention that pelvic tilt also may affect labor progress. (page 598)

5. The nurse should explain that frequency refers to the elapsed time from the start of one contraction to the start of the next; duration is the elapsed time from the start to the end of one contraction. (page 599)

6. During labor, gastric motility and absorption decrease and gastric emptying time increases. Consequently, a client in labor may vomit food consumed up to 24 hours before labor began. Thus, the nurse advises Penny not to eat solid foods to prevent the risk of aspiration if an emergency arises and she needs general anesthesia. Because gastrointestinal absorption of fluids is not altered, Penny is permitted to sip fluids. (pages 603 and 604)

Multiple choice

7. (a). This describes the nesting instinct. (page 585)

8. (d) (page 586)

9. (d) (page 587)

10. (c) The trochanter is the bony process of the femur. (page 584)

Study questions

11. *Nitrazine test.* Vaginal discharge is tested with nitrazine paper to determine its pH, thereby distinguishing between SROM and urinary incontinence caused by uterine pressure on the bladder. With SROM, the nitrazine paper turns blue because amniotic fluid is alkaline.
Ferning test. This test identifies amniotic fluid in a dried smear of vaginal fluid by its unique fernlike pattern, as seen under a microscope.
Pooling. This refers to direct observation of fluid pooled within the vagina. The test is performed by sterile speculum examination; if the membranes have ruptured, the examiner observes fluid leaking into the vagina. (page 586)

12. Cardinal movements occur in the following chronological order:
(1) descent
(2) flexion
(3) internal rotation
(4) extension
(5) external rotation
(6) expulsion (page 587)

13. Fetal descent results from one or more of the following forces: contraction of the abdominal muscles, pressure from amniotic fluid, direct fundal pressure on the fetus, or extension and straightening of the fetus. (page 587)

14. The sutures function to permit fetal skull bones to overlap as they press together during the fetus's passage through the pelvis; and they aid in identifying fetal position during labor. (page 594)

15. Vertex is the usual fetal attitude in the uterus. The head is flexed so that the chin rests against the chest, the legs and arms are folded in front of the body, and the back is curved forward slightly. (page 594)

16. Predisposing factors in a fetal shoulder presentation include placenta previa, neoplasm, fetal anomalies, hydramnios, preterm labor, uterine atony, multiple gestation, and premature artificial rupture of the membranes. (page 594)

17. The three planes of the true pelvis are the pelvic inlet, the midpelvis, and the pelvic outlet. These planes are significant because diameters measured within them indicate the amount of space available for the fetus during delivery. (pages 598 and 600)

18. The fetus is at 0 station when the largest diameter of the presenting part is level with the ischial spines. Palpation of the ischial spines indicates progressive fetal descent, suggesting a successful vaginal delivery. (pages 597, 598, and 601)

19. The three phases of a uterine contraction are the increment, the acme, and the decrement. (page 591)

20. Three conditions that cause placental malfunction are placenta previa, abruptio placentae, and uteroplacental insufficiency. (page 602)

21. Contractions during the first stage of labor increase systolic blood pressure by about 10 mm Hg and diastolic pressure by 5 to 10 mm Hg. Because of this fluctuating increase, blood pressure readings between contractions are most reliable. (page 603)

22. Reduced sensory perceptions during labor may impair the ability to sense bladder fullness and the urge to void; compression of the ureters by the enlarged uterus also may impede urine flow. Consequently, urinary stasis may occur; an overextended bladder may impede fetal descent. (page 604)

Fill in the blank

23. downward movement (page 587)

24. floating (page 587)

25. extension (page 589)

26. restitution (page 589)

27. anteroposterior (page 589)

28. expulsion (page 589)

29. third (page 591)

30. 7.35; 7.25 (page 605)

31. 7.2 (page 605)

Matching terms and definitions

32. (1) a; (2) e; (3) g; (4) b; (5) h; (6) c; (7) f; (8) d (page 585)

Labeling illustrations

33. For the locations of the fetal skull bones, fontanels, and sutures, see the illustration on text page 592.

34. The correct fetal presentations and positions are as follows:
Illustration a: frank breech presentation
Illustration b: right occiput posterior (ROP) position
Illustration c: left occiput anterior (LOA) position
Illustration d: brow presentation
Illustration e: face presentation (pages 595, 596, and 597)

ANSWERS FOR CHAPTER 25 • FETAL ASSESSMENT

Page numbers in parentheses refer to textbook pages.

Clinical simulations

1. Use of epidural anesthesia during labor can impair normal vasoconstriction of maternal peripheral blood vessels. As these vessels dilate and hold more blood, hypotension develops and less blood returns to the heart. This decreases maternal cardiac output and impairs blood flow to the uterus, which may compromise fetal oxygenation and cause prolonged FHR deceleration. (page 610)

2. Late decelerations indicate uteroplacental insufficiency and may lead to fetal hypoxia and acidosis unless the underlying cause is corrected. As prescribed, the nurse should discontinue the oxytocin, turn Marianne onto her left side to increase placental perfusion and decrease contraction frequency, increase the I.V. fluid rate to enhance intravascular volume and placental perfusion, and administer oxygen by mask at 7 liters/minute. Notify the physician immediately. Explain these interventions to Marianne and her family, stressing that they are essential to fetal health. (page 619)

Multiple choice

3. (d) (page 616)

4. (b) (page 610)

Study questions

5. Any factor that decreases maternal cardiac output reduces placental blood flow. Such factors include maternal position, uterine contractions, placental surface area and diffusion distance, anesthetics, maternal hypertension or hypotension, and cord compression. (page 609)

6. The autonomic nervous system receives information about blood pressure and oxygen status from chemoreceptors (sensory nerve cells) and baroreceptors (pressure-sensitive nerve endings in the walls of large systemic arteries); this helps the fetal central nervous system stabilize blood pressure. Chemoreceptors detect even minute changes in tissue oxygenation, triggering the sympathetic nervous system to boost the FHR so that more blood circulates to the affected area, increasing tissue oxygenation. As a result, fetal blood pressure increases. Baroreceptors are highly sensitive to blood pressure increases; in response to an increase, they signal the parasympathetic nervous system to decrease FHR rapidly. As FHR declines, so do fetal cardiac output and blood pressure. (page 610)

7. A supine maternal position during labor reduces uterine blood flow. As the gravid uterus compresses the vena cava and hinders blood return to the heart, the client may develop supine hypotensive syndrome. In this syndrome, blood pressure and cardiac output decrease, reducing blood flow to the uterus and decreasing placental perfusion. Or the aorta may become compressed, reducing blood

flow to the uterus. In either case, uteroplacental perfusion is compromised, leading to fetal hypoxia. (page 609)

8. The nurse may assess FHR with a fetoscope, an ultrasound stethoscope, or an electronic fetal monitor. (page 611)

9. The nurse must monitor the uterine contraction pattern as closely as the FHR to help detect fetal distress. Normally, as the uterus contracts, oxygenation to the uterus and fetus decreases; as the uterus relaxes, oxygenation is restored. Contractions occurring at 3-minute intervals dilate the cervix most effectively and allow sufficient time for reoxygenation of the fetus and uterine muscle. Increased uterine activity may progress to hyperstimulation, which reduces placental perfusion and can lead to fetal distress. (page 614)

10. The nurse assesses uterine contractions through manual palpation, an external tocodynamometer (external electronic monitoring), or an internal intrauterine pressure catheter (internal electronic monitoring). According to most experts, the internal intrauterine pressure catheter yields the most accurate results. (page 615)

11. Signs of fetal hypoxia that may appear on a fetal monitor strip are persistent baseline tachycardia, bradycardia, decreased variability, and late decelerations. (pages 617 and 618)

12. Two causes of decreased FHR variability that have a gradual onset and may pose a serious threat to the fetus are fetal hypoxia and acidosis. Initially, the fetus may react to hypoxemia with increased variability. As a continued oxygen decrease progresses to hypoxia, the fetus attempts to increase oxygenation and the heart rate accelerates; baseline tachycardia with decreased or absent variability results. Over time, lack of oxygen harms the fetal CNS. If this cycle continues, acidosis and direct fetal cardiac depression develop. Baseline bradycardia may arise as the fetus nears death. (pages 617 and 618)

13. A variable deceleration FHR pattern has an abrupt onset and rapid recovery; takes a variable waveform shape, possibly resembling the letter U, V, or W; and commonly is accompanied by an FHR that decreases to 60 beats/minute. (page 621)

14. The fetal scalp stimulation test, in which gentle digital pressure or an Allis clamp is applied to the fetal scalp, normally provokes a positive (or reactive) response by the fetus, indicating fetal stability and well-being. In a positive response, FHR accelerates by 15 beats/minute for at least 15 seconds. (page 623)

15. The three general categories to document are assessment findings, procedures, and interventions. Specific items to document include:
    - the frequency, duration, and intensity of uterine contractions
    - the baseline FHR
    - the continuous range of the FHR pattern
    - any tachycardia or bradycardia, including the times at which these occurred

- any long-term or short-term variability
- any accelerations
- any decelerations, noting whether these are early, late, variable, or prolonged
- appropriate nursing interventions that were performed, based on monitor readings
- the outcome of the interventions (pages 623 and 624)

Fill in the blank

16. baseline FHR (page 616)

17. movement (page 616)

True or false

18. True (page 617)

19. True (page 617)

20. False (page 617)

21. False (page 619)

22. True (page 619)

23. False (page 619)

Matching terms and definitions

24. (1) h; (2) f; (3) c; (4) b; (5) g; (6) a; (7) e; (8) d; (9) i (page 609)

Page numbers in parentheses refer to textbook pages.

Clinical simulations

1. The nurse should be concerned about Linda's excessive anxiety because it may prolong labor and increase pain perception. An anxious client has increased cardiac output and blood pressure and possibly an increased risk of:
   - impaired gastrointestinal function, which can reduce gastric emptying and raise the aspiration risk
   - decreased urinary function, which may lead to oliguria
   - higher epinephrine and norepinephrine levels, which can prolong labor, cause hyperventilation, and result in fetal hypoxia
   - increased plasma cortisol levels, which may lengthen labor and decrease uterine activity.

   Also, because Linda is unprepared, she is more susceptible to the fear-tension-pain cycle. In this cycle, fear and anxiety increase muscle tension, resulting in vasospasm-induced ischemia, which causes pain. This in turn increases anxiety. Nursing interventions for Linda seek to reduce anxiety, thus decreasing her blood pressure and heart rate, allowing greater energy production for effective uterine contractions, and reducing muscle tension and the heightened pain perception such tension causes. The nurse's presence, confidence, attention, and concern can help control Linda's anxiety. Reassure, encourage, and praise her throughout labor. As labor progresses, keep her informed, teach and reinforce coping strategies, and assure her that labor is progressing normally. If she becomes discouraged or frustrated, reassure her and help her to choose an alternate method of comfort promotion. Helping Dan also may reduce Linda's anxiety. Support Dan's efforts to comfort her, and offer instructions and help as appropriate. (pages 630 and 633)

2. Labor pain is altering Carol's behavioral responses. (page 630)

3. A posterior fetal position typically causes severe sacral pain. If this is determined to be the cause of Cindy's pain, the nurse should attempt to help rotate the presenting part to an anterior position by having Cindy:
   - assume an all-fours position and rock her pelvis
   - combine kneeling or squatting with pelvic rocking to promote fetal rotation, unless these positions are uncomfortable or tiring
   - straddle a chair to remain upright
   - use a squatting or side-lying position for pushing during the second stage of labor. (page 634)

4. Denise is experiencing hypotensive crisis. The nurse should turn Denise to the left lateral position to increase uterine perfusion; infuse I.V. fluid rapidly and administer oxygen by mask, as prescribed; elevate Denise's legs to increase venous return; notify the anesthesiologist; be prepared to administer a vasopressor, as prescribed; stay

with Denise; and monitor blood pressure and fetal heart rate frequently. (page 641)

Multiple choice

5. (b) Endorphin release is central to another theory of pain transmission—the endogenous opiate theory. (page 635)

6. (a) (page 638)

7. (d) I.V. analgesia must be instilled slowly, for at least a full minute, during the peak of a contraction. (page 640)

Study questions

8. Techniques used to promote relaxation during labor include distraction, progressive muscle relaxation, yawning, controlled breathing, imagery, touch, and music therapy. (page 634)

9. During stage 1, pain results mainly from cervical effacement and dilation. During the latent phase (cervical dilation of 0 to 3 cm), clients typically describe the pain as an ache or discomfort. During active labor (4 to 7 cm dilation), pain becomes moderately sharp. During the transitional phase (7 to 10 cm dilation), pain is severe, sharp, and cramping. Throughout most of the stage 1, pain centers around the pelvic girdle; during late stage 1, it spreads to the upper legs and perineum. During stage 2, pain results from friction between the fetus and birth canal and from pressure on the perineum, bladder, bowel, and uterine ligaments. In the early part of stage 2, pain is located in the upper legs and perineum; during late stage 2, intense pain develops at the perineum. During stage 3, pain results from ischemia caused by contraction of uterine blood vessels. As in late stage 2, it is located at the perineum. (pages 627 to 629)

10. Factors that can affect a client's perception of and ability to cope with labor pain include parity, fetal size and position, certain medical procedures, anxiety, fatigue, education, culture, and coping mechanisms. (pages 628 and 630)

11. Medical procedures or actions that can increase client discomfort during labor include conducting a vaginal examination on a supine client, using a tight abdominal belt to secure a fetal monitor, forbidding a client to change positions or walk, and administering an enema. (pages 628 and 630)

12. Before administering pain-relief agents, the nurse must consider fetal age and development, because an immature fetus has a diminished ability to metabolize analgesic agents; and fetal heart rate, because this is a primary indicator of fetal well-being. (page 632)

13. Promoting hygiene can increase client comfort by boosting self-esteem, providing distraction, removing additional sources of discomfort, and blocking pain perception. Nursing interventions that promote hygiene during labor include providing showers and bathing, ensuring perineal care, providing oral hygiene, and frequently changing soiled linens and clothing. (page 633)

14. *Analgesia* refers to pain reduction without loss of consciousness. Although the client who has received an analgesic may continue to perceive pain, the pain typically is more tolerable because the analgesic affects the peripheral nervous system (by relaxing muscles and increasing blood flow) and the central nervous system. *Anesthesia* refers to partial or complete loss of sensation, sometimes with loss of consciousness. It affects the entire body or only a region of it, blocking conduction of impulses along pain pathways to the brain. (page 637)

15. The nurse educator should describe all options for analgesia and anesthesia, including administration route, degree and timing of pain relief, impact on labor and the fetus, potential adverse drug reactions, and effectiveness. Also explain how a particular anesthetic or analgesic may interfere with the client's active labor participation, and describe the immediate and prolonged effects of pharmacologic agents on the neonate. (page 637)

16. Regional anesthesia techniques commonly used during vaginal delivery include epidural block, pudendal block, and local infiltration. (pages 640 to 642)

17. The epidural block—the most commonly used pain-relief method during labor—is achieved through injection of a local anesthetic into the epidural space (third to fifth lumbar inner space).
Advantages. The epidural block reduces pain continuously throughout the first and second stages. Although it causes the pelvis and legs to feel heavy, the client retains some ability to move and bear down. Also, this method can be used if complications arise and cesarean delivery is necessary.
Disadvantages. Skilled anesthesia personnel must be on hand to monitor the client and fetus. Also, an epidural block may prolong labor, cause voiding difficulty, increase oxygen use, and increase the likelihood of forceps delivery because of the client's diminished bearing-down efforts. The epidural block requires much skill to achieve complete and effective anesthesia; improper infusion may cause areas of unanesthetized tissue, ineffective anesthesia, or inadvertent spinal anesthesia.
Adverse effects. Maternal hypotension may result from sympathetic blockade, which can cause vasodilation, peripheral resistance loss, and central nervous system toxicity. The client may feel chilled from peripheral temperature changes and may experience postpartal urine retention necessitating catheterization. (page 641)

18. The nurse should document any comfort measures that were taken and their effectiveness, the analgesic agent administered and its effectiveness, vital signs, any changes in uterine contractions after analgesia administration, and changes in fetal heart rate after analgesic administration. (page 645)

Fill in the blank

19. anxiety; muscle tension (page 634)

20. pain (page 634)

ANSWERS FOR CHAPTER 27 • THE FIRST STAGE OF LABOR

Page numbers in parentheses refer to textbook pages.

Clinical simulations

1. No. The nurse should assume Mrs. Byrd is in false labor because she lacks evidence of cervical change and has mild, irregular contractions that diminish with walking. (page 654)

2. The nurse should suggest appropriate comfort measures and explain medical orders. Suggest that Ms. Byrd take a warm tub bath or shower assisted by a family member to ease discomfort, drink warm milk or herbal tea, and recline semi-upright with pillows under her knees to promote rest. Encourage her to drink clear liquids and eat light meals rich in carbohydrates. Suggest that her support person provide massage to promote comfort. Instruct her to return to the health care facility if her membranes rupture, if bleeding occurs, if her contractions become regular and more intense, if she shows signs of infection, or if fetal movements change dramatically. (page 660)

3. Ms. Nordstrom's health history findings should be prioritized as follows: (a) 10; (b) 11; (c) 5; (d) 4; (e) 3; (f) 8; (g) 12; (h) 6; (i) 1; (j) 7; (k) 2; (l) 9 (page 651)

4. Tests missing from this list are a complete blood count (CBC), urinalysis, and gonorrhea culture. A CBC screens for anemia, infection, blood dyscrasias, and bleeding problems. Urinalysis screens for pregnancy-induced hypertension, renal disease, and infection. Gonorrhea culture detects gonorrhea. (page 664)

5. Leopold's maneuvers help determine fetal lie, presentation, and position. They help detect potential problems, such as breech presentation, that require physician or nurse-midwife evaluation, as well as help anticipate the course of labor. (page 657)

6. These findings indicate breech presentation. (page 656)

7. The nurse should assess Jeanette's vital signs (blood pressure, pulse, and respirations) at least every 30 minutes. If her membranes are intact, measure her temperature every 4 hours; if her membranes have ruptured, measure her temperature every 2 hours while checking her pulse. Assess uterine contractions at least every 30 minutes or according to facility policy. Assess fetal heart tones every 15 minutes or according to facility policy. (pages 666 and 667)

8. For Mary's husband, the nurse can promote confidence in his ability to support Mary; welcome him on admission; include him in Mary's history and physical assessment; evaluate goals for his involvement in childbirth; assess his physical and emotional needs and plan ways to address them during labor; reduce his anxiety and awkward feelings by showing concern for his interest and participa-

tion in childbirth; make him feel important to Mary's comfort and support; direct care and support measures if he is hesitant or unprepared; suggest appropriate times for him to take a break to eat, rest, or attend to personal hygiene; help him listen to fetal heart tones whenever desired; inform him of routine changes in fetal heart rate patterns and their significance; assure him that frequent monitoring does not signal an impending problem; and keep him involved if a crisis arises during labor. If he has been prepared for labor and childbirth, also reinforce his knowledge of conscious relaxation and breathing techniques, promote his interaction, and foster successful sharing of the experience.

For Mary's mother, be sensitive to how she may react to unfamiliar and perhaps frightening medical technology, regularly inform her of Mary's progress, and advise her about necessary medical treatments or procedures.

For Mary's son, introduce yourself, be aware that his response to childbirth depends mainly on his maturity and interest, and maintain a calm, matter-of-fact attitude to reassure him that everything is proceeding normally. (page 675)

Study questions

9. For a new client, assessment focuses on determining the imminence of birth and establishing fetal stability. (page 650)

10. To increase client comfort when performing a vaginal examination, t he nurse should have the client empty her bladder beforehand; maintain her dignity by helping her into a comfortable lithotomy position and draping her; talk to her and maintain eye contact during the examination; suggest conscious relaxation techniques to help her relax her vaginal muscles; cover her with the bed sheet, if she desires; and provide perineal hygiene and change the disposable pad under her buttocks, as needed. (pages 660, 668, and 669)

11. Conditions that can mimic true labor include false labor, urinary tract infections, and abruptio placentae. (page 654)

12. True labor is distinguished from false labor (Braxton Hicks contractions) by evaluation of contractions, pain, fetal movement, fetal descent, show, and cervical changes. In true labor, contractions are regular and rhythmic; pain moves from the back to the front of the abdomen; fetal movement is unchanged; fetal descent progresses; show consists of pinkish mucus, possibly with the mucus plug from the cervix; and the cervix undergoes progressive effacement and dilation. In false labor, contractions are irregular; mild discomfort or pressure occurs in the abdomen and groin; fetal movement may intensify; fetal descent remains unchanged; no show appears; and the cervix does not progress after 1 to 2 hours. (page 654)

13. The nurse should question the client about the amount, color, and odor of the amniotic fluid as well as the time of rupture. (page 654)

14. To promote comfort for the client in active labor, the nurse should create a supportive atmosphere, promote good positioning and walking, maintain hygiene, conserve energy, provide pain-relief measures, promote rest and effective breathing, provide appropri-

ate teaching, integrate her cultural beliefs and practices into nursing care, and relieve pain. These measures are important because they reduce maternal anxiety and help prevent fetal stress resulting from uterine dysfunction and intrauterine hypoxia—conditions associated with increased maternal anxiety. (page 670)

15. The nurse should document the date, time, examination findings, examiner's name, and the procedures that were performed, such as amniotomy and fetal scalp electrode placement. Also record fetal heart tones in response to the procedures, the uterine contraction pattern, the client's vital signs, and her response to the procedures. (pages 660 and 679)

Fill in the blank

16. contractions; dilation (page 648)

17. false labor (page 654)

True or false

18. False (page 659)

19. True (page 659)

20. False (page 659)

21. False (page 657)

22. True (page 657)

Matching terms and definitions

23. (1) m; (2) g; (3) b; (4) a; (5) k; (6) i; (7) f; (8) e; (9) c; (10) d (page 649)

ANSWERS FOR CHAPTER 28 ◆ THE SECOND STAGE OF LABOR

Page numbers in parentheses refer to textbook pages.

Clinical simulations

1. If the client has a strong urge to bear down before the cervix dilates completely, edema and tissue damage may occur, impeding fetal descent. To help Ms. Madison avoid bearing down, the nurse should assist her onto her forearms and knees, a position that decreases the urge to bear down by relieving pressure on the rectum. Instruct her to blow or pant through each contraction until her cervix has receded completely. To increase her comfort in this position, raise the head of the bed and place several pillows under her arms. (page 684)

2. Advantages of the lateral recumbent position include the following:
   - It corrects or avoids adverse hemodynamic effects of the lithotomy position.
   - It places less tension on the perineum.
   - It may help rotate an occiput posterior presentation.
   - It may help relieve shoulder dystocia.
   - It may increase comfort and rest between contractions because contractions are less frequent.
   - It promotes maximum uterine blood flow and fetal oxygenation.
   - It helps control the delivery.

   Disadvantages of the lateral recumbent position include the following:
   - It may impede bearing-down efforts.
   - It requires someone to hold the client's leg up for delivery.
   - It may be awkward for the birth attendant.
   - It may impair the birth attendant's ability to see and interact with the client.
   - It may complicate episiotomy repair or use of forceps.
   - It may make fetal heart tones harder to hear. (page 690)

3. The nurse should assign Todd an Apgar score of 6—2 points for heart rate, 1 point each for respiratory effort, muscle tone, reflex irritability, and color. Because this score indicates mild respiratory, metabolic, or neurologic depression, the nurse should stimulate Todd's breathing by gently but firmly slapping the soles of his feet or rubbing his spine or sternum. As prescribed, administer 100% oxygen via bag and face mask. Observe him continuously for improvement in respirations, heart rate, color, tone, and reflexes and assign another Apgar score at 5 minutes. (page 695)

4. Ms. Albrecht should mention that an episiotomy may help prevent damage to the anal sphincter and rectal mucosa, allow for easier repair and better healing than a spontaneous laceration, prevent trauma to the fetus's head, and prevent serious damage to pelvic floor muscles. (pages 692 and 693)

Study questions

5. Signs of the second stage include an increasing urge to push, possibly accompanied by perineal bulging in a multiparous client; an increase in bloody show, caused by greater cervical dilation; grunting; gaping of the anus; involuntary defecation; bulging of the vaginal introitus; spontaneous rupture of the membranes; and abrupt onset of early decelerations, possibly caused by fetal head compression. (pages 682 and 683)

6. The first phase of the second stage is completed when the presenting part reaches the pelvic floor. The second phase ends when the neonate is delivered. During the first phase, the client may not feel a strong urge to bear down; typically, these urges are short, manageable, and occur at the peak of each contraction. During the second phase, the client typically feels an uncontrollable urge to push and her bearing-down efforts are most effective at expelling the fetus. (page 683)

7. Fetal factors that may affect duration of the second stage include physical condition, size, station, position, molding, rotation, and rate of descent. Maternal factors include parity, labor position, fatigue level, age, degree of expulsive efforts, strength of uterine contractions, size and shape of the bony pelvis, resistance or relaxation of soft tissues, and such obstetric interventions as anesthesia and episiotomy. (page 683)

8. Variations in FHR patterns during the second stage may result from umbilical cord compression, fetal descent, and maternal bearing-down efforts. (page 685)

9. Adverse outcomes of a prolonged second stage include infant mortality, postpartal maternal hemorrhage, neonatal seizures, puerperal febrile morbidity, and changes in neonatal acid-base status. (page 684)

10. To assign an Apgar score, the nurse should assess the neonate's heart rate, respirations, muscle tone, reflex irritability, and color. (page 695)

Fill in the blank

11. cervical dilation; delivery of the neonate (page 683)

12. 1; 30 (page 685)

13. fetal distress (page 685)

14. 2 hours (page 684)

ANSWERS FOR CHAPTER 29 ◆ THE THIRD AND FOURTH STAGES OF LABOR

Page numbers in parentheses refer to textbook pages.

Clinical simulations

1. The nurse should expect the placenta to have calcifications, discolorations, malformations, cysts, or umbilical cord abnormalities. Such findings provide information about the neonate's status, helping to explain fetal distress and low birth weight. (pages 707 and 708)

2. Factors that place Judy at high risk for postpartal hemorrhage include her previous history of heavy postpartal bleeding, delivery of a large-for-gestational-age neonate, hydramnios, extended stimulation of labor with oxytocin, traumatic delivery, and grand multiparous status. (pages 707 and 710)

3. The nurse should suspect uterine atony, clot retention, or a full bladder. Appropriate nursing measures include massaging the fundus until it becomes firm and clots are expressed; reassessing the fundus at least every 5 minutes; urging Sharon to void; encouraging her to initiate breast-feeding (if desired); and administering oxytocin, if prescribed. (page 714)

4. The nurse should suspect a vaginal hematoma, which requires immediate attention by the physician or nurse-midwife. (pages 713, 715, and 716)

5. Ms. Peng's behavior, which consists of classic maternal responses, demonstrates positive mother-infant bonding. She is holding her son in the en face position, which reflects an attempt to establish his reality and health. (page 717)

Multiple choice

6. (b) (page 705)

7. (c) (page 705)

8. (d). Fewer than three umbilical vessels correlates with various congenital anomalies, such as cardiac and renal anomalies. (pages 708 and 709)

Study questions

9. The third stage of labor typically lasts from a few minutes to 30 minutes. (page 705)

10. The normal signs of placental separation are a sudden gush or trickle of blood from the vagina, increased umbilical cord length at the vaginal introitus, a change in uterine shape from discoid to globular, and a change in the position of the uterus to a location at or above the umbilicus. (page 707)

11. The two mechanisms of placental expulsion are the Duncan and Schultze mechanisms. The Duncan mechanism occurs when the dark, rough, maternal side of the placenta is delivered first. The

Schultze mechanism occurs when the glistening fetal side of the placenta appears first. (page 707)

12. When assisting with episiotomy repair, the nurse should provide adequate light, suture material, a local anesthesia kit (if necessary), and support. Assess for an intact suture line, and note the degree of swelling, oozing, or discoloration caused by bruising or hematoma formation. (page 707)

13. Immediate physiologic changes associated with postpartal hemorrhage include an increasing pulse rate, followed by increased respirations and reduced blood pressure. Postpartal hemorrhage typically results from uterine atony, excessive blood loss during placental separation and delivery, or perineal lacerations. (page 707)

14. After delivery, the nurse should assess the neonate's respiratory and cardiovascular status, assign an Apgar score, and maintain adequate body temperature. (pages 710 and 712)

15. Thermoregulation is crucial to the neonate because the metabolic rate increases to produce heat if hypothermia occurs. This can cause respiratory distress, which can progress to metabolic acidosis and require aggressive treatment.

    To help prevent hypothermia, the nurse should dry the neonate thoroughly after delivery, promote skin-to-skin contact with the mother, wrap the neonate in warm blankets or place under a radiant warmer, and cover the neonate's head with a stockinet cap or a plastic bunting covering. (page 712)

16. Nursing interventions during the fourth stage of labor include maintaining appropriate maternal positioning and activity, preventing hemorrhage, maintaining hygiene and comfort, maintaining fluid balance, meeting nutritional needs, and promoting parent-infant bonding. (page 717)

17. During the fourth stage of labor, the nurse should assess the client at least every 15 minutes. The assessment should include vital signs, fundus, lochia, perineum, leg pain, and tremors. Also assess the client's comfort level; recovery from analgesia or anesthesia; level of fatigue, hunger, and thirst; and response to the neonate. (pages 713, 714, and 716)

18. Engrossment refers to positive bonding between father and child. It is characterized by tactile, visual, and verbal activities that the father directs at the neonate. Typically, the father touches the neonate's skin, looks closely at the neonate, and expresses feelings of elation. (page 717)

19. During the fourth stage of labor, common causes of an elevated maternal temperature are dehydration, fatigue, and infection. (page 714)

ANSWERS FOR CHAPTER 30 ◆ FAMILY SUPPORT DURING THE INTRAPARTAL PERIOD

Page numbers in parentheses refer to textbook pages.

Clinical simulations

1. Like any client who has a constant companion during labor, Lisa may have a shorter labor and significantly fewer obstetric complications; experience decreased pain and anxiety; have less need for labor-inducing drugs and anesthetics; have more positive feelings about the childbirth experience; show better coping behaviors; and receive comfort, reassurance, and assistance with pain control techniques from her support person. (page 728)

2. Ms. Klein's response is an example of perceived support—her belief that support is available if she needs it; such support may be more important to her than actual support. Ms. Klein perceives support because she feels that Justin cares about her and will help if asked. (Received support, in contrast, occurs when one person takes specific actions to support another to communicate a caring attitude.) (page 728)

3. David can help Betsy by providing a calming influence, reducing her loneliness, providing helpful distractions, and communicating her needs to health care professionals. (page 729)

4. Once it becomes obvious to the nurse that the visitors are distracting or annoying Rosalind, the nurse should ask that all visitors except Steve leave the room. As an impartial client advocate who probably will not see the visitors again, the nurse is in a better position than Rosalind to take responsibility for this decision. (page 733)

5. Based on the 1987 study by Kintz, these supportive nursing behaviors should be ranked as follows:
   (a) 6; (b); (c) 7; (d) 1; (e) 4; (f) 5; (g) 2 (page 729)

Study questions

6. Support refers to feelings of affection, trust, and affirmation and the sharing of advice, information, and time between people to help an individual gain, regain, or use personal strength during difficult or challenging situations. (pages 727 and 728)

7. Common sources of support for the client in labor include the client's partner, family members, friends, and health care professionals. (page 727)

8. The nurse must tailor specific strategies for client and family support to the client's individual needs because each client's pain tolerance, coping skills, and cultural beliefs differ. Although nearly all clients experience pain and anxiety during labor and delivery, the degree of pain experienced, the ability to cope with pain, verbal and nonverbal responses to pain, and the cultural beliefs that affect these responses vary. A client who experiences more pain during

labor usually needs more support than one who experiences less pain. (page 728)

9. Touch can convey sensitivity to the client's need for comfort, pain relief, and alleviation of fear and anxiety. The nurse can encourage a support person to show caring through touch by using such actions as holding the client's hand or stroking her face. (page 729)

10. Many Korean-American clients prefer a middle-aged woman as a support person. The woman need not be a relative but must have many sons and much experience in delivering children. Typically, these clients do not want men or childless women in the labor and delivery area.

    In contrast, many Mexican-American clients prefer a female relative or friend as a support person; all female relatives may play a prominent role in support for these clients, who regard the extended family as an important part of the childbirth experience. (page 730)

11. Birth culture is a set of beliefs, values, and norms of action surrounding the birth process that are shared to various degrees by members of a cultural or ethnic group. It informs members of the group about the nature of conception, the proper conditions for procreation and childbearing, the mechanism of pregnancy and labor, and the rules and rationales of prenatal and postnatal behavior. Birth culture may influence a client's diet, her response to labor, preferred positions for childbirth, activity restrictions, and family members' roles during childbirth. (page 732)

12. Nursing assessment of the primary support person should focus on the support person's knowledge of how to assist the client during labor and on personal concerns about labor. (page 731)

ANSWERS FOR CHAPTER 31 • HIGH-RISK INTRAPARTAL CLIENTS

Page numbers in parentheses refer to textbook pages.

Clinical simulations

1. A mature, healthy client such as Courtney has many of the same intrapartal nursing needs as a younger client. The nurse should anticipate that Courtney's greatest needs will be psychosocial because the admission assessment shows an uncomplicated, closely monitored pregnancy with no evidence of pregnancy-induced hypertension (PIH), intrauterine growth retardation, placenta previa, premature rupture of the membranes (PROM), or premature labor. However, because of the initial pelvic findings and the tendency of the mature client to develop labor dysfunction, the nurse should monitor Courtney's contraction pattern, which can affect the efficiency of contractions, and should assess fetal position, which can help determine labor duration. (pages 741 and 751)

2. Factors that contributed to Courtney's arrested labor include her age and such fetal factors as malposition and a minus two station. Lack of fetal descent suggests cephalopelvic disproportion (CPD), which also contributes to labor dysfunction. Labor dysfunction is relatively common in mature clients due to decreased efficiency of the aging myometrium or increased incidence of CPD, leiomyomata, and fetal malposition (such as occiput posterior presentation). (page 751)

3. If Courtney's contractions become less efficient or cease and cervical dilation or fetal descent are arrested, the nurse should expect to assist with I.V. fluids, oxytocin augmentation, and continuous electronic fetal monitoring (EFM). (page 751)

4. The increased incidence of vacuum extraction in mature clients may stem from decreased efficiency of the aging myometrium, decreased maternal stamina, and increased use of epidural anesthesia. After delivery, the nurse should assess Courtney for postpartal hemorrhage related to uterine atony—a possible sequela of oxytocin augmentation after a difficult labor. (page 754)

5. The nurse should suspect diabetic ketoacidosis (DKA) as the cause of Ms. Simone's signs and symptoms. This condition, which can be triggered by the stress of labor in a pregnant client with diabetes, is a form of acidosis accompanied by ketone accumulation in the blood. DKA constitutes an obstetric emergency because it can lead to coma and death unless treated promptly; it also can cause fetal acidosis and fetal distress. Until prompt treatment restores maternal homeostasis, Ms. Simone is at risk for diabetic complications and her fetus is at risk for intrauterine death. (pages 752 and 753)

6. The nurse should summon the obstetrician and other members of the health care team, including the diabetologist and internist, as required. To help confirm DKA, obtain arterial blood gas (ABG) lev-

els, as prescribed. Use a reagent strip to evaluate Ms. Simone's urine for ketones and use a reflectometer to monitor blood for a glucose test. Send for baseline laboratory studies, such as electrolyte and serum blood glucose levels. Record hourly fluid intake and output on a flowsheet. Document blood glucose and urine acetone levels, laboratory test results for ABG levels and electrolyte studies, maternal vital signs, and fetal heart rate (FHR). As prescribed, start an I.V. line with an isotonic solution. Monitor Ms. Simone's cardiac status with a bedside ECG monitor, if possible; check for signs of hyperkalemia, which can precipitate cardiac arrhythmias. Attempt to maintain serum potassium in the 4 to 5 mEq/liter range. Expect to draw blood to check serum potassium levels every hour. After fluid replacement has been initiated, administer short-acting regular insulin, as prescribed. Monitor blood glucose levels every hour. Administer I.V. solutions that contain glucose only after the blood glucose level ranges from 150 to 200 mg. Monitor the FHR and variability continuously. (page 753)

7. Mrs. Caruthers's history and physical findings strongly suggest PIH. Specific suggestive findings include her elevated blood pressure, edema, headache, blurred vision, proteinuria, brisk reflexes, and lack of prenatal care. Potential maternal complications of PIH include insufficient perfusion of vital organs, seizures, hypertonic uterine activity, abruptio placentae, and preterm labor. Potential fetal or neonatal complications include prematurity, toxicity (if Mrs. Caruthers receives magnesium sulfate), intrauterine growth retardation resulting from poor uteroplacental insufficiency, and complications associated with low birth weight, including increased fetal distress, and meconium aspiration. (pages 741 to 743 and pages 746 to 749)

8. Goals of nursing care for Mrs. Caruthers include taking seizure precautions to avoid general injury and reduce nervous system irritability; helping to prevent or treat seizures with medications, as prescribed; assessing maternal and fetal response to treatment; and assessing for related complications, such as pulmonary edema or disseminated intravascular coagulation. (pages 752 to 754)

9. Many factors can predispose a client to intrapartal infection. Because Candy is an adolescent, she is at increased risk for anemia, sexually transmitted diseases, and preterm labor—all of which predispose her to intrapartal infection. Her prolonged PROM also contributes to the risk of infection. (pages 742 and 743)

10. Nursing care for Candy's intrapartal infection involves immediate administration of I.V. fluids to improve hydration, reduce fever, and prevent exhaustion. The nurse should use external EFM to avoid further contamination of the fetus. Expect to assist in collecting blood or vaginal cultures to identify the infecting organism; also expect to administer a prescribed broad-spectrum I.V. antibiotic (unless contraindicated by any allergies). Carefully assess maternal and fetal response to infection treatments.

    Prepare for labor induction or augmentation with oxytocin, as prescribed, to shorten the time to delivery. Also limit the number of vaginal examinations and provide meticulous perineal care. Anticipate spontaneous vaginal delivery, depending on the severity of the infection and maternal and fetal tolerance for labor. Be sure to address Candy's adolescent psychosocial needs.

Notify the neonatal team to ensure that they are ready for Candy's potentially ill neonate. The neonate will be preterm and thus at increased risk for sepsis; lung problems, such as respiratory distress syndrome, also are likely. If Candy received adequate antibiotics for sepsis during labor, her neonate is less likely to have respiratory depression at birth; if not, the neonate may require resuscitation. Coordinate family care and convey all pertinent information to the nursery and postpartal teams. After delivery, collect specimens for cultures from Candy, the neonate and possibly the placenta, as prescribed. (pages 750 and 755)

Study questions

11. During labor, even a client with minimal activity limitations during pregnancy may experience sudden worsening of the disease. Labor can cause sudden, profound cardiovascular changes. For instance, pain and increased venous blood return from the uterus boost cardiac output 20% during each contraction. Mean arterial pressure rises and is followed by reflex bradycardia. Uterine contractions can compress the aorta and iliac arteries, forcing more blood to the upper torso and head. (page 742)

12. For this client, bearing down during the second stage of labor can reduce venous blood flow to the heart by increasing thoracic pressure. When the client stops bearing down, cardiac output and blood pressure increase rapidly, putting extra stress on the heart. (page 754)

13. Psychosocial problems during labor and delivery are especially common among adolescents because of unfamiliar surroundings, a sense of isolation, heightened fears and fantasies about labor and delivery, and the forthcoming responsibilities of motherhood. (page 739)

14. Substance abuse can cause problems that may affect the antepartal period and lead to intrapartal problems. For example, severe nutritional deficiencies and sexually transmitted diseases, which are common among women who abuse drugs, compromise fetal health. Substance abuse can cause social isolation, which can affect the client's ability to cope with labor. Use of nonsterile needles can cause maternal infection or embolization, which can affect maternal and fetal health. Cocaine use during pregnancy causes maternal and fetal vasoconstriction, tachycardia, and elevated blood pressure. These effects decrease blood flow to the fetus and can stimulate uterine contractions. Cocaine abuse also increases the risk of preterm labor, delivery of a low-birth-weight or small for-gestational-age neonate, and abruptio placentae.

15. The client with PIH typically complains of multisystemic symptoms because PIH reduces perfusion to nearly all tissues. Headache and mental confusion reflect poor cerebral perfusion and may precede seizures. Visual disturbances, such as scotomata, result from retinal arterial spasm and edema. Complaints of epigastric pain or stomach upset may signal hepatic distention, a warning sign of impending preeclampsia. Tightness and intermittent numbness in the hands indicate ulnar nerve compression from edema. Excessive weight gain over 1 week usually relates to edema of the face, hands, and feet. (page 746)

16. To diagnose PIH, the client's prenatal blood pressure is compared to her current reading. In preeclampsia, blood pressure increases by at least 30 mm Hg systolic or 15 mm Hg diastolic from baseline values. If prenatal blood pressure is unknown, a reading of 140/90 mm Hg after 20 weeks' gestation suggests preeclampsia. In severe preeclampsia, blood pressure measures 160 mm Hg systolic or 110 mm Hg or more diastolic and significant edema and proteinuria are present. (page 747)

17. Magnesium sulfate is the treatment of choice for seizure prevention. It prevents seizures by depressing neuromuscular transmission, which diminishes hyperactive reflexes. It also reduces cerebral edema and intracranial pressure, which cause mild vasodilation. (page 753)

18. Signs of magnesium sulfate toxicity include hypotension, respiratory paralysis, and reduced reflexes. Calcium gluconate is prescribed for a magnesium sulfate overdose. (pages 743 and 754)

19. The nurse must address the needs of the family of the high-risk intrapartal client because family members are likely to experience extreme anxiety for the client and the fetus. They may feel left out, isolated from the client, and intimidated by the setting, equipment, and staff. If they focus on the seriousness of the client's condition, they may lose sight of the impending celebration of birth. (page 759)

ANSWERS FOR CHAPTER 32 • SPECIAL OBSTETRIC PROCEDURES

Page numbers in parentheses refer to textbook pages.

Clinical simulations

1. The potential risks of cesarean delivery include preterm birth, anesthesia risk, aspiration pneumonia, injury to urinary tract organs or the bowels, bowel obstruction, wound dehiscence leading to evisceration, infection, hemorrhage, and thromboemboli. (page 778)

2. The physician would explain that in an internal podalic version, rapid delivery of a second twin in a breech position is attempted. After administering an anesthetic agent, the clinician reaches one hand through the vagina and cervix and into the uterus, grasps the fetus's legs, and performs an assisted breech delivery. The physician would tell Roberta and Steve that if this procedure fails, emergency cesarean delivery would be needed.
Discussing the risks and complications of an internal version, the physician would mention uterine trauma; lacerations of the perineum, vagina, or cervix; postpartal hemorrhage; and fetal injury. (pages 768, 769, 770, and 777)

3. To help alleviate Roberta's fears and provide psychological support for her and Steve, the nurse can provide them with basic information about the procedure, explaining each step. Reassure them that it is relatively safe for the fetuses and, whenever possible, offer choices to involve them in decisions. Be prepared to listen and respond to their concerns. Make sure Roberta has given written consent. (page 782)

4. The nurse should inform Roberta that she may be able to have a vaginal birth after cesarean (VBAC) delivery. Tell her that VBAC has advantages and disadvantages compared to repeated cesarean deliveries. Mention such advantages as the family experience of a normal childbirth, reduced risk of infection and death, shorter recovery time, and lower cost. Mention such potential disadvantages as the risk of uterine rupture. However, inform Roberta that physicians disagree about the extent of this and other suggested disadvantages, and point out that among clients who have had low-transverse cesarean delivery and wish to attempt vaginal delivery, about 70% have a successful vaginal delivery. (pages 773 and 774)

5. The client who has had a cesarean delivery through a transverse incision made in the lower uterine segment may have a successful vaginal delivery with a subsequent pregnancy. (page 774)

6. The nurse should explain that in vacuum extraction, the physician applies a suction cup device called a ventouse to the fetus's scalp, creates suction by removing the air mechanically, and pulls to help deliver the fetus. Mention that a vacuum extraction decreases delivery time and does not require additional space inside the vaginal canal as does forceps delivery. (pages 773 and 774)

7. The nurse-midwife should inform the Bachs that if labor does not follow amniotomy closely, infection may result (from prolonged premature rupture of the membranes). Mention that if amniotomy does not induce labor, Greta will require oxytocin infusion; if this fails, cesarean delivery may be required. (page 771)

8. The nurse might suggest that Ms. Marks maintain a knee-to-chest position for 15 minutes, three times a day for 7 days, to help the fetus shift to a cephalic presentation. (page 770)

9. An episiotomy helps shorten the second stage of labor, especially when evidence of fetal distress exists and an assisted forceps delivery is required. Tucker-McLean forceps help prevent head trauma in preterm neonates. (pages 772 and 774)

Multiple choice

10. (c) (page 780)

11. (d) (pages 774 and 775)

12. (b) (page 772)

Study questions

13. The transverse lower uterine segment incision requires extra time, limits the area for extension if more maneuvering space is needed to extract the fetus, and may extend laterally into major uterine vessels. (page 776)

14. External version is used to rotate the fetus from a breech or shoulder presentation to a cephalic presentation. To minimize potential complications, the procedure should be performed late in the third trimester, before engagement of the presenting part, only if amniotic fluid is sufficient, and only if the membranes are intact. (page 768)

15. The two major considerations in labor induction are fetal age and cervical readiness. The fetus must be fully mature and the cervix must be likely to dilate and efface in response to induction. (page 770)

16. Excess fluid can cause water intoxication in a client undergoing oxytocin labor induction. Oxytocin has a potent antidiuretic action, which can decrease the free water clearance of the kidneys, in turn reducing urine production. (page 770)

17. Amniotomy improves the efficiency of uterine contractions because amniotic fluid release decreases uterine volume, causing the fetal presenting part to serve as a more efficient dilating wedge. Also, it may shorten labor when the cervix is soft, dilated, anteriorly positioned, and effaced to some degree; allows earlier detection of meconium-stained amniotic fluid, which can result in fetal pneumonia; and permits internal probe monitoring of the fetus and uterus. (page 771)

18. During a forceps delivery, the nurse must check the fetal heart rate (FHR) after the physician has applied the forceps but has not yet ap-

plied traction to the fetus; a decrease in FHR could signal cord compression. Also assess the client's vital signs and comfort level. Immediately after forceps delivery, assess the neonate for cerebral trauma. Observe the client closely for signs of tissue trauma, such as excessive bleeding, pain, hematoma, and cervical or vaginal lacerations. Inform nursery personnel and postpartal caregivers that the neonate was delivered by forceps. (page 780)

True or false

19. False (page 768)

20. True (page 770)

21. False (page 773)

22. False (page 776)

23. False (page 778)

24. True (page 775)

ANSWERS FOR CHAPTER 33 • INTRAPARTAL COMPLICATIONS

Page numbers in parentheses refer to textbook pages.

Clinical simulations

1. Ms. Nacione is experiencing hypotonic uterine dysfunction. This pattern typically occurs during the active phase of labor. (pages 788 and 789)

2. The client's presenting signs and symptoms suggest abruptio placentae. (page 793)

3. In a case of unexpected fetal death, the nurse should provide the same physical care as to any other client in labor as well as assist and comfort the client and family, allowing them to grieve. Monitor Ms. Paulson's coagulation studies, as prescribed, because she may be at risk for disseminated intravascular coagulation. After she has delivered the dead fetus, give her and her husband the chance to see and hold the child if they wish. Wrap the child in a blanket and prepare the Paulsons for its appearance. Give them as much time as they wish to spend with their child. Offer to provide a lock of hair, footprints, and bracelets; even if the Paulsons decline, gather these items in case they change their minds. A photograph of the child also may be appropriate. If the Paulsons want to have their child baptized, the nurse can perform this rite, regardless of religion. Avoid reassuring platitudes that prevent the Paulsons from expressing their feelings. (page 804)

Multiple choice

4. (d) (page 790)

5. (b) (page 794)

6. (a). Attempting to replace the cord may traumatize the cord, stop blood flow to the fetus, or cause an intrauterine infection. (page 795)

Study questions

7. Potential fetal effects of dysfunctional labor include hypoxia, asphyxia, and physical injuries sustained during descent. (page 790)

8. For a client who is experiencing uterine inversion, the nurse should monitor the client's blood loss, fluid status, and vital signs to detect shock. Expect to administer blood transfusions and be prepared to assist other members of the health care team with measures that attempt to reverse the uterus. (pages 798 and 800)

9. If a precipitate delivery is imminent, the nurse should help the client and anyone with her to remain calm and summon additional professional help immediately. Never leave the client alone. Gather the necessary equipment, and prepare the client for a calm, controlled delivery using the most sterile technique possible under the circumstances. To promote a good delivery outcome, try to gain her confidence and cooperation. (page 791)

10. The cardinal sign of placenta previa is painless vaginal bleeding after the twentieth week of pregnancy. (page 792)

11. Conditions that may contribute to abruptio placentae include maternal hypertension, a short umbilical cord that places traction on the placenta, trauma, a uterine anomaly or tumor, sudden decompression of the uterus, pressure on the vena cava from the enlarged uterus, and dietary deficiencies. (page 792)

12. Signs of fetal distress include an abnormal fetal heart rate pattern, a change in fetal activity, and meconium-stained or yellow amniotic fluid after rupture of the membranes. (page 796)

13. Appropriate nursing actions to take in response to fetal distress include repositioning the client in the lateral or knee-chest position to improve maternal-fetal circulation; administering oxygen by face mask at 8 to 10 liters/minute to improve fetal oxygenation; notifying the physician and the surgical team to direct management of this emergency; assisting with I.V. fluid administration to manage maternal hypovolemia or hypotension; discontinuing any oxytocin immediately to improve uteroplacental perfusion; remaining calm and purposeful when caring for the client to help prevent undue fear and anxiety, which could adversely affect uteroplacental perfusion; and providing explanations and reassurance to the client to help her gain control and cooperate fully. (page 796)

14. The nurse should provide the client and family with updated information to allay their anxiety, assess their coping mechanisms, determine the strength of their support systems, help family members express their fears and concerns, and share information to clarify misconceptions and to make them feel involved. (page 801)

Fill in the blank

15. hypotonic; hypertonic (page 788)

16. progression; 3 (page 789)

17. placenta previa (page 792)

18. abruptio placentae (page 792)

19. 1,000; hydramnios (page 794)

20. breech (page 796)

ANSWERS FOR CHAPTER 34 • NEONATAL ADAPTATION

Page numbers in parentheses refer to textbook pages.

Clinical simulations

1. The condition that the Mardsleys have noticed is acrocyanosis. The nurse should explain that this common neonatal phenomenon results from vasomotor instability, capillary stasis, and high hemoglobin levels. Reassure them that acrocyanosis does not indicate a breathing problem; such a problem would manifest as an overall blue tinge to the skin and mucous membranes (central cyanosis), reflecting poor gas exchange. (page 825)

2. The nurse should inform Ms. Althus that high maternal estrogen levels may cause transient side effects in a neonate. Explain that the blood she found in her daughter's diaper reflects pseudomenstruation, a mucoid or blood-tinged vaginal discharge seen in some female neonates that results from the sudden drop in hormone levels after birth. Tell Ms. Althus that both male and female neonates may have breast hypertrophy with or without witch's milk—a thin, watery secretion similar to colostrum. Reassure her that these problems are clinically insignificant and will resolve spontaneously when the influence of maternal hormones subsides. (page 825)

3. The pediatrician diagnoses pathologic jaundice because of the early onset and marked degree of Brittany's bilirubin elevation. Pathologic jaundice stems from such conditions as blood group or blood type incompatibilities; hepatic, biliary, or metabolic abnormalities; or infection. If Brittany is not treated and her unconjugated serum bilirubin level reaches 20 mg/dl or higher, she may develop bilirubin encephalopathy, a life-threatening condition characterized by bilirubin deposition in the basal ganglia of the brain. (page 817)

4. The nurse should encourage Ms. Zanelli to breast-feed her son at this time. In most cases, as in Tanya's, feedings should begin as soon as the neonate is stable physiologically and shows adequate coordination of the sucking and swallowing reflexes. An extended delay before feedings may deplete the neonate's limited glycogen reserves, already taxed by the increased energy demands of the transitional period. Glycogen depletion may result in hypoglycemia, which poses a threat to the glucose-dependent brain. (pages 819 and 820)

Multiple choice

5. (c) (page 814)

6. (b) (pages 815 and 816)

7. (d). Whether the neonate can produce heat by shivering remains unknown; even if shivering does occur, it is not a major heat source. (page 824)

8. (a) (pages 816 and 817)

Study questions

9. Functional closure of the foramen ovale refers to cessation of blood flow, caused by pressure changes within the left atrium and increased systemic resistance, rendering the structure nonfunctional. Anatomic closure occurs several months later with structural obliteration from constriction or tissue growth. (page 812)

10. The mechanical forces that result in fluid removal from the neonate's lungs are chest compression, elastic recoil, and glossopharyngeal (frog) breathing. Chest compression occurs as the neonate squeezes through the birth canal, forcing out approximately one third of the lung fluid through the nose and mouth. Elastic recoil pulls air into the lungs as the neonate's chest clears the birth canal. Glossopharyngeal breathing, which involves involuntary muscle contractions, pulls additional air into the lungs. (pages 814 and 815)

11. Conditions necessary to maintain neonatal respiratory function within the first 24 hours are a patent airway, a functioning respiratory center, intact nerves from the brain to the chest muscles, and adequate calories to supply energy for the labor of breathing. (page 816)

12. For several days after birth, the gastrointestinal tract lacks the bacterial action to synthesize adequate vitamin K. (Vitamin K catalyzes synthesis of prothrombin by the liver, thereby activating four coagulation factors in the blood.) To prevent hemorrhagic disease, all neonates receive a prophylactic injection of vitamin K soon after delivery. (page 817)

13. The neonate's neurologic system regulates adaptation by stimulating initial respirations, maintaining acid-base balance, and controlling body temperature. (page 822)

14. Crucial neonatal reflexes include feeding reflexes, protective reflexes, postural reflexes, and social reflexes. (page 822)

15. Mechanisms of neonatal heat loss include evaporation, conduction, radiation, and convection.
Evaporative heat loss occurs when fluids turn to vapor in dry air. To minimize the pronounced evaporative heat loss accompanying delivery, the nurse should dry the neonate immediately and discard the wet towels. *Conductive heat loss* occurs when the skin directly contacts a cooler object. To prevent such heat loss, make sure all metal surfaces on which the neonate will be placed are padded. *Radiant heat loss* results when a cooler solid surface not in direct contact with the neonate pulls heat away from the neonate. To minimize radiant heat loss, make sure a thermoplastic heat shield is used to surround the neonate in the incubator. *Convection* causes heat loss from the body surface to cooler surrounding air, especially in drafty environments. To avoid convective heat loss, protect the neonate from drafts caused by air conditioning ducts or windows. (page 824)

16. The neonate's early weight decrease results from loss of fluid through urine, feces, and insensible losses; through intake restric-

tions related to small gastric capacity; and through an increased metabolic rate. (page 819)

17. Vision, hearing, touch, taste, and smell are present at birth. Using these senses, the neonate perceives, interacts with, modifies, and learns from the environment. Combined with the neonate's attractive physical features, these sensory capacities play a key role in parent-neonate attachment. (page 826)

18. This series of characteristics is called the periods of neonatal reactivity. Familiarity with these periods enables the nurse to recognize the neonate's normal characteristics and thus assess the neonate more skillfully, plan more effective neonatal care, and help promote parent-neonate interaction. (pages 827 and 828)

19. The first period of reactivity is the optimal time for promoting mother-infant bonding. Beginning just after birth, it lasts roughly 30 minutes. It is characterized by intense activity and awareness of external stimuli. The neonate is alert and attentive to the environment and may exhibit vigorous activity and crying, rapid respiratory and heart rates, and a strong desire to suckle. Gradually, the neonate becomes less alert and active and falls asleep. (page 827)

20. Conditions that can lead to hypoglycemia in the normal neonate include cold stress, delayed feeding, metabolic abnormalities, and sepsis. (page 822)

21. The sensory, cerebellar, and extrapyramidal pathways are the first nerve pathways to develop. Early development of the sensory pathways accounts for the neonate's strong sense of hearing, touch, and smell. The cerebellum governs gross voluntary movement and helps maintain equilibrium. The extrapyramidal tract controls reflexive gross motor movement and postural adjustment by regulating reciprocal flexion and extension of muscle groups, thus maintaining smooth, coordinated movements. (page 822)

Fill in the blank

22. transient tachypnea (page 815)

23. nonshivering thermogenesis; brown fat (page 824)

Identifying anatomic structures

24. See *Tracing neonatal circulation,* text page 813.

ANSWERS FOR CHAPTER 35 • NEONATAL ASSESSMENT

Page numbers in parentheses refer to textbook pages.

Clinical simulations

1. Large for gestational age (LGA) is a term used to describe a neonate whose birth weight exceeds the ninetieth percentile for gestational age on the Colorado intrauterine growth chart. Antepartal history findings that might predict LGA status include a fundal height that is disproportionate to gestational weeks and maternal diabetes mellitus or an elevated maternal serum glucose level. (pages 833 to 835)

2. *Katy's physical maturity scores:*
   - skin: 2
   - lanugo: 2
   - plantar surface: 4
   - breast: 3
   - eye and ear: 2
   - genitalia: 3

   Subtotal = 16

   Katy's neuromuscular maturity scores:
   - posture: 3
   - square window: 3
   - arm recoil: 4
   - popliteal angle: 4
   - scarf sign: 2
   - heel to ear: 3

   Subtotal = 19

   Katy's maturity rating score (sum of subtotals) = 35. Katy's gestational age = 38 weeks.

   According to the Ballard tool, Katy is a full-term neonate; her gestational age is 38 weeks, not 36 weeks as indicated by the date of her mother's last menstrual period. Her weight falls below the tenth percentile for gestational age on the Colorado intrauterine growth chart; therefore, she is classified as small for gestational age (SGA).

   Katy's case demonstrates that unless weight and gestational age are plotted, a neonate's estimated gestational age may be erroneous, and a birth-weight variation, such as Katy's SGA status, might go undetected. Early identification of gestational-age and birth-weight variations improves a neonate's chance for survival by allowing the health care team to anticipate the perinatal problems associated with such variations. (pages 840, 842, and 843).

Maturity rating													
Score	–10	–5	0	5	10	15	20	25	30	35	40	45	50
Weeks	20	22	24	26	28	30	32	34	36	38	40	42	44

Multiple choice

3. (c) The nurse should combine overlapping portions of the various assessments to help conserve the neonate's energy. (pages 832, 834, and 842)

4. (c) (page 857)

5. (d) (page 850)

6. (b) (page 846)

Study questions

7. The nurse should check the maternal antepartal and intrapartal records for any problems that the client might have experienced during pregnancy. By detecting such problems, the health care team can anticipate potential perinatal problems more accurately. (page 834)

8. Immediate assessment of the neonate (determination of the Apgar score) includes skin color, heart rate, respiratory rate, muscle tone, and reflex irritability. (page 834)

9. A neonate's vital signs, state of alertness, and responsiveness to external stimuli change with the period of reactivity. The nurse must be able to recognize the characteristics of each period and interpret assessment findings with these characteristics in mind. Stay alert for deviations from the findings normally associated with each period; such deviations may signify a disorder. (page 835)

10. (a) Normal
(b) Abnormal. Possible causes: prematurity, respiratory distress, sepsis, transient tachypnea
(c) Abnormal. Possible causes: hypothermia, poor peripheral perfusion, prematurity, infection
(d) Normal
(e) Normal
(f) Normal (pages 836 and 837)

11. Signs of labored breathing include uneven chest expansion, nasal flaring, visible chest retractions, expiratory grunts, and inspiratory stridor. (page 837)

12. The Dubowitz tool and the Ballard tool are the most commonly used gestational-age assessment tools. The Dubowitz tool measures 11 external and 10 neurologic criteria. The Ballard tool, an abbreviated version of the Dubowitz tool, measures 7 physical maturity and 6 neuromuscular maturity criteria. Refined periodically in response to current research, the Ballard tool can be used at any time after delivery. The Dubowitz tool, in contrast, should be delayed until after 24 hours, to eliminate external influences on the neonate's neurologic functioning. (pages 839 and 841)

13. A cephalhematoma is a collection of blood between the skull and periosteum that does not cross suture lines. Commonly caused by forceps trauma, the condition may last up to 8 weeks.
Caput succedaneum refers to localized pitting edema of the scalp,

possibly crossing suture lines. It results from pressure on the fetal occiput, as during extended labor. (page 857)

14. (page 851)

NORMAL RESPONSE	REFLEX	TESTING METHOD
a. Neonate extends extremities on the side to which the head is turned and flexes extremities on the opposite side.	Fencing (tonic neck) reflex	With a swift motion, turn the neonate's head to either side.
b. Neonate makes walking motions with both feet.	Stepping (automatic walking) reflex	Hold the neonate upright and touch one foot lightly to a flat surface.
c. Neonate extends and abducts all extremities bilaterally and symmetrically; forms a "C" shape with the thumb and forefinger; and adducts then reflexes, extremities.	Moro reflex	Suddenly but gently drop the neonate's head backward (relative to the trunk).
d. Neonate sucks on a finger forcefully and rhythmically; sucking is coordinated with swallowing.	Sucking reflex	Place a finger in the neonate's mouth.
e. Neonate hyperextends the toes, dorsiflexes the great toe, and fans the toes outward	Babinski reflex	Stroke one side of the neonate's foot upward from the heel across the ball of the foot.

15. Responses evaluated on the Brazelton neonatal behavioral assessment scale include habituation, orientation, motor maturity, variations, self-quieting ability, and social behaviors. (page 852)

16. Parents who observe the behavioral assessment can learn firsthand about their neonate's behavioral and interactive capacities. Some experts believe that such observation improves parent-child interaction, promotes more appropriate parental responses to neonatal behavioral cues, and makes parent-neonate interaction more mutual. The nurse also can use this opportunity to assess the parents' behavior and determine the quality of parent-neonate interaction. (pages 852 and 868)

Fill in the blank

17. 2 (page 836)

18. head (page 836)

19. neurologic (page 839)

20. 45 to 53; 32 to 35 (page 836)

Matching terms and definitions

21. (1) c; (2) h; (3) b; (4) e; (5) i; (6) f; (7) a; (8) g; (9) d (page 855)

ANSWERS FOR CHAPTER 36 ♦ NURSING CARE OF THE NORMAL NEONATE

Page numbers in parentheses refer to textbook pages.

Clinical simulations

1. The nurse should keep in mind that even if a neonate is placed under a radiant warmer and dried to reduce heat loss immediately after delivery, wide temperature fluctuations are common during the first few hours after birth. If Jason has been kept in an open warmer for 2 to 3 hours and his core (rectal) temperature is above 96.8° F (36° C), the nurse may wrap him in a blanket and place him in an open, clear basinette for a visit with his mother. To ensure a neutral thermal environment, the nurse should monitor Jason's skin temperature, which should measure 32° to 32.9° F (0° to 0.5° C) below the core temperature. (page 874)

2. Yes, an initial feeding is appropriate. For a bottle-fed neonate, the first feeding should not be delayed more than 6 hours after birth. During the first feeding, the nurse should assess Emily's sucking ability and observe how well she coordinates the sucking, swallowing, and gag reflexes. Immediately after the feeding, check for salivation, mucus production, aspiration, and regurgitation. (pages 875 and 876)

3. The nurse should instruct Ms. Dunbar to compare Steven's fluid intake to his urine output to ensure adequate hydration. Mention that he should receive 140 to 160 ml/kg/day of fluid. Inform her that the breast-fed neonate usually voids at least six times a day, and tell her to call the physician if Steven does not saturate his diaper moderately at least five times a day. Teach Ms. Dunbar to inspect Steven's urine color, which should be clear and amber. Instruct her to watch for signs of dehydration, such as decreased skin turgor, a depressed anterior fontanel, and sunken eye orbits. Stress that she should report such signs to her health care provider immediately. (page 875 and 877)

4. To ensure environmental home safety for eonates, Ms. Briggs should instruct the clients to provide for room lighting that is strong enough to allow accurate observation of the neonate's skin color and respiratory effort, have a clock within easy view, minimize noise in the neonate's room, keep a consistent room temperature, and maintain humidity at 35% to 60%. She should advise them to protect the neonate from drafts and to keep window shades drawn to minimize neonatal heat loss. To promote the neonate's digestion, she should urge them to position the neonate on the abdomen or right side after a feeding, to elevate the head of the bed to help prevent aspiration, and to avoid placing pillows, toys, or stuffed animals in the neonate's bed because these items could cause suffocation if they fall onto the neonate's head.

   Because a neonate can move on a flat surface, increasing the risk of falling, Ms. Briggs should caution clients never to look away or leave the neonate unattended and to keep the crib sides up and in the locked position before leaving the bedside. She should emphasize that when traveling with the neonate, they should place the neonate in an infant car seat and apply the seat belt. (pages 884, 885, and 887)

Multiple choice

5. (c) (page 872)

6. (b) (page 874)

7. (a) (page 875)

Study questions

8. To detect instability, the nurse must evaluate the neonate's heart rate and rhythm, respiratory rate and rhythm, skin color, cry, response to stimuli, alertness level and irritability level. (page 872)

9. A bulb syringe is preferred because a sterile suction catheter may cause apnea, reflex bradycardia, cardiopulmonary arrest, or laryngospasm. (page 873)

10. Potential signs of neonatal respiratory distress include dusky or cyanotic skin, grunting, nasal flaring, and crackles or rhonchi. (page 874)

11. The neonate's first stool consists of meconium, a thick, dark green, sticky, odorless material. Once feeding patterns are established, stool color and consistency change. Transitional stools appear; these stools are thinner, lighter green, and seedier than meconium. After 2 or 3 days, stools take on distinctive characteristics that vary with the feeding method. The stool of a breast-fed neonate is looser and paler yellow than that of a formula-fed neonate. Also, the breast-fed neonate typically passes two to ten stools daily; the formula-fed neonate, one stool daily or every other day. (page 877)

12. Nonspecific signs that suggest neonatal infection include a high, low, or unstable body temperature; a weak or high-pitched cry; pallor; cyanosis; feeding problems or fatigue after feedings; diminished peripheral perfusion causing reduced skin temperature;sudden onset of apneic or bradycardia episodes; and jaundice. (page 879)

13. The nurse should serve as a caregiver role model for the parents and reinforce their caregiving behaviors. When the neonate rooms-in with the client, the parents can observe the nurse caring for the neonate, then practice such care in a supervised setting as the nurse offers positive reinforcement and constructive criticism. This promotes the parents' self-confidence and can strengthen the parent-infant bond. (page 885)

14. Typically, the parents' attitude toward circumcision is influenced by religious beliefs, the perception that circumcision is a sign of manhood, and the fear that an uncircumcised male will be stigmatized. (page 888)

ANSWERS FOR CHAPTER 37 • INFANT NUTRITION

Page numbers in parentheses refer to textbook pages.

Clinical simulations

1. No contraindications exist for breast-feeding a healthy, full-term neonate immediately after delivery. Therefore, the nurse should encourage Amy to begin breast-feeding at this time. Early breast-feeding has many benefits. For example, during the first 30 minutes or so after birth, the neonate is highly responsive and eager to suck. Amy's breasts may be soft and easy to manipulate now, promoting proper attachment; also, her daughter's licking or nuzzling motions, which indicate readiness to feed, will help stimulate Amy's prolactin production. Immediate breast-feeding also offers the chance for intimate contact that can enhance mother-infant bonding and have a positive psychological effect on the parents. (page 910)

2. The nurse should encourage Dave to provide physical support (such as helping with housework or other children), verbal reinforcement (such as ensuring Amy that breast-feeding is progressing well), and psychological support or sensitivity to Amy's feelings. Urge him to help Amy rest when she is establishing her milk supply and to prevent visitors from overwhelming her in the early postpartal days. (page 918)

3. The nurse should explain that milk supply increases in response to demand; therefore, the more milk Amy's daughter requires through frequent breast-feeding, the more milk Amy will produce. Tell Amy she can expect to breast-feed every 2 to 3 hours while building up her milk supply. Advise her to check the number of wet diapers to gauge her daughter's milk intake: An infant who wets 10 to 12 diapers in a 24-hour period is getting adequate intake. Steady weight gain and contentedness after feedings are other indications of adequate intake. Encourage Amy to breast-feed long enough for her daughter to receive the rich, more filling hindmilk; this takes about 15 minutes on each breast as Amy establishes her milk supply. (pages 903 and 914)

4. No. The nurse should inform Amy that giving supplemental bottled fluids to a breast-feeding neonate is an outmoded, unscientific practice. Besides causing nipple confusion, supplemental bottles given in the early weeks of breast-feeding may interfere with the fragile dynamics of milk supply and demand. Advise Amy to avoid giving supplemental bottles until her milk supply is well established, which usually takes 4 to 6 weeks. (page 915)

5. The nurse should caution Ms. Johnson not to feed her son cow's milk until he is at least 6 months old. Point out that cow's milk contains hard-to-digest protein curd and that intake of whole milk can result in a high renal solute load, which may cause fluid imbalance. Explain that the high mineral content of whole milk coupled with

the neonate's low glomerular filtration rate can cause excessive fluid excretion, increasing her son's fluid needs even more. Also mention that cow's milk has poorly absorbed butterfat and can cause gastrointestinal bleeding if consumed in large amounts with little solid food. (pages 894, 895, and 907)

6. The nurse should instruct Ms. Johnson not to give her son solid foods until he is 3 months old. Point out that before then, he is not ready to ingest solid foods because he has limited synthesis of the starch-splitting salivary enzyme ptyalin and lacks pancreatic amylase, which restricts digestion of complex starches found in solid food. Tell Ms. Johnson that the extrusion reflex, in which the tongue pushes out food placed on it, does not diminish until approximately age 4 months. Inform her that an infant under 3 months lacks the tongue motion needed to pass solids from the front to the back of the mouth; this may lead to choking. (pages 894 and 895)

7. Maternal factors to assess include positioning of the bottle and neonate during feeding and proper adjustment of feeding technique in response to the neonate's cues; also assess Ms. Ettinger's breasts for signs of engorgement. Neonatal factors to assess for include excessive drooling, coughing, gagging, or respiratory distress during feeding; amount of formula the neonate takes; mucus in regurgitated matter; how readily the neonate burps; signs of lactose intolerance; and presence of circumoral cyanosis. (page 909)

8. The nurse should assess the consistency of Ms. Poirier's breasts, nipple condition, and the sensations she experiences during feeding. Also assess the neonate's sucking reflex, signs of lactose intolerance, proper mother and neonate positioning, and the neonate's attachment to the breast. (page 908)

9. The nurse should teach Ms. Morasco about the upright, across-the-lap, and upright-in-the-lap burping positions. In the upright position, Ms. Morasco places her neonate lengthwise, with his head on her shoulder, then pats or rubs his back with one hand while supporting him with the other. In the across-the-lap position, she places him across her lap, holds his head with one hand, then rubs or pats his back with the other. In the upright-in-the-lap position, she places him upright on her lap and holds his head from the front with one hand while patting or rubbing his back with the other hand; to help bring up air, she rocks him back and forth gently.

Also instruct Ms. Morasco to burp her son after every ounce of formula and again at the end of the feeding. Advise her to place a towel or cloth diaper in front of him to protect her clothing because he may expel milk along with air. (pages 913 and 921)

10. The nurse can advise Ms. Morasco to feed her son on a flexible demand schedule, not a rigid regimen. Inform her that formula-fed infants may awaken for feedings as often as every 2 hours or as infrequently as every 5 hours; many feed satisfactorily on a 3- to 4-hour schedule. If Ms. Morasco worries that her son is not getting enough nourishment, reassure her that a neonate's initial feeding pattern does not necessarily reflect the pattern that will emerge later. (page 921)

Multiple choice

11. (c). These women more readily incorporate siblings into the feeding experience. (page 903)

12. (b) (page 903)

Study questions

13. The three basic nutrients are carbohydrates, proteins, and fats. Carbohydrates should serve as the infant's main source of calories. Proteins promote cellular growth and maintenance, aid metabolism, and contribute to many protective substances. Fats provide a concentrated energy storage form, transport essential nutrients (such as fatty acids needed for neurologic growth and development), and insulate vital organs. (page 894)

14. At the start of a feeding, foremilk is released. This thin, watery substance is low in calories but abundant in water-soluble vitamins; it accounts for about 60% of the total volume of a feeding. Next, whole milk is released. The hindmilk is available 10 to 15 minutes after initial let-down; it has the highest concentration of calories for satisfying hunger between feedings. (page 902)

15. Signs of lactose intolerance include abdominal cramps and distention and diarrhea. Lactose intolerance is caused by absence of the enzyme lactase in the border of the intestinal villi; lactase breaks down lactose, the major carbohydrate in milk. A common treatment for lactose intolerance is the use of a soy-based formula, which provides corn syrup solids and sucrose as the primary carbohydrates. (page 908)

16. The nurse should include such topics as initiating breast-feeding, correct infant attachment and positioning, removing the infant from the breast, burping the infant, establishing a breast-feeding pattern, night feedings, coping with growth spurts, expressing milk, nipple and breast care, supplementary bottles, ensuring adequate maternal fluid and food intake, drug use while breast-feeding, and family support. (pages 910 to 919)

17. Basic methods of infant formula preparation include the aseptic method, the terminal method, the one-bottle method, and the clean method. (pages 920 and 921)

18. Colostrum contains high concentrations of protein, fat-soluble vitamins, minerals, and immunoglobulins (which function as antibodies). Its advantages include its laxative effect, which promotes early passage of meconium; also, the low colostrum volumes produced do not tax the neonate's limited gastric capacity or cause fluid overload. (page 902)

19. Infant growth spurts occur at ages 10 to 14 days, 6 weeks, 3 to 4 months, and 6 months. (page 914)

Fill in the blank

20. 150 (page 894)

21. weight; length; head circumference (page 895)

22. 1 year (page 895)

23. 180 (page 906)

Chronological order

24. (a) 3; (b) 5; (c) 2; (d) 4; (e) 1 (page 900)

Matching terms and definitions

25. (1) a, c, f, g; (2) b, d, e

Values clarification

26. through **32.** No correct answers exist.

ANSWERS FOR CHAPTER 38 ◆ HIGH-RISK NEONATES

Page numbers in parentheses refer to textbook pages.

Clinical simulations

1. Like any neonate of a client with gestational diabetes, Bennett has an increased risk of asphyxia, infection, respiratory distress, severe hypoglycemia, hypocalcemia, hyperbilirubinemia, polycythemia, and death. (page 938)

2. When assessing Bennett for hypoglycemia, the nurse should stay alert for apnea, bradycardia, seizures, irregular respirations, cyanosis, irritability, listlessness, lethargy, tremors, feeding problems, vomiting, hypotonia, and a high-pitched cry. In a preterm neonate such as Bennett, the physician confirms hypoglycemia from two serum glucose values below 25 mg/dl during the first 72 hours. (pages 938 and 951)

3. General nursing measures during phototherapy focus on maintaining body temperature; timing care properly to avoid unnecessary stress; and assessing oral intake, urine output, and stools. The nurse should observe Jonathan closely for respiratory compromise because of his increased risk for asphyxia and respiratory distress resulting from prematurity and hyperbilirubinemia.
Specific nursing actions that will help ensure Jonathan's safety during phototherapy include the following:
   - Place an opaque mask over his eyes to help prevent retinal damage, and observe for signs of pressure caused by the mask.
   - Cover the genitals with a mask or small diaper.
   - Turn off the phototherapy lights for 2 to 5 minutes at least every 8 hours to assess Jonathan's eyes for irritation and help him establish a normal sleep-awake pattern.
   - Monitor the number and consistency of stools, and clean his buttocks after each stool to help maintain skin integrity.
   - Check his serum bilirubin level every 4 to 8 hours to determine the effectiveness of phototherapy.
   - Estimate fluid losses and assess for dehydration. (page 969)

4. To identify signs of HIV infection, the nurse should assess Maura for facial dysmorphism, hepatosplenomegaly, interstitial pneumonia, subtle neurologic abnormalities, behavioral changes, and recurrent infections. (page 953)

Multiple choice

5. (c) (pages 927 and 929)

6. (d) (page 930)

7. (a) (page 930)

Study questions

8. The major goals of neonatal intensive care are to avert or minimize complications, subject the neonate to as little stress as possible, and further parent-infant bonding. (page 932)

9. Although meningomyelocele sometimes can be corrected by surgery, the child may be left with paralysis, necessitating costly, lifelong care. In some cases, the physician or parents may believe that the poor quality of life that awaits the child justifies withholding treatment; the expense of lifelong care is a complicating issue. (page 933)

10. The most common problems seen in the NICU are prematurity and its sequelae, congenital heart defects, and congenital anomalies requiring emergency surgery. (page 933)

11. Complications of prolonged neonatal asphyxia include cerebral hypoxia, seizures, intraventricular hemorrhage, renal failure, necrotizing enterocolitis, and metabolic imbalances. Without immediate resuscitation, a neonate with prolonged asphyxia will die. (page 933)

12. Congenital anomalies that pose a threat to the neonate's life and warrant immediate intervention include tracheoesophageal malformations, diaphragmatic hernia, choanal atresia, omphalocele, gastroschisis, meningomyelocele, encephalocele, and imperforate anus. (page 942)

13. The congenital heart defects described are (a) patent ductus arteriosus, (b) tetralogy of Fallot, (c) atrial septal defect, (d) transposition of the great vessels, and (e) coarctation of the aorta. (pages 946 and 947)

14. Depending on the neonate's condition and response to each resuscitative measure, neonatal resuscitation typically involves some combination of free-flow oxygen, positive-pressure ventilation, closed-chest cardiac massage, gastric decompression, emergency drugs, and endotracheal intubation. (page 957)

15. To promote parent-infant bonding, the nurse should encourage the parents to contribute to their child's environment by attaching a small family item, such as a family photograph, to the neonate's bed. Allow the parents to touch and hold their child whenever possible and provide them with simple caregiving tasks, such as diaper changes. Point out how their child responds to their presence, voice, and touch, and show them how to offer appropriate sensory stimulation so that they can take an active role in their child's development. (page 971)

16. Findings that reflect fluid volume excess are (a), (d), (f), (h), and (i). Findings that reflect fluid volume deficit are (b), (c), (e), and (g). (page 967)

Fill in the blank

17. 37 (page 934)

18. 42 (page 934)

19. tenth (page 935)

20. ninetieth (page 936)

True or false

21. False (page 937)

22. False (page 937)

23. True (page 947)

Chronological order

24. (a) 6; (b) 2; (c) 7; (d) 3; (e) 4; (f) 8; (g) 1; (h) 5 (pages 958 to 960)

Matching terms and definitions

25. (1) a, b, c, e, f, i, k, m, n, p; (2) c, d, g, k, o; (3) c, d, h, j, k, m; (4) g, k, m (pages 934 and 935)

ANSWERS FOR CHAPTER 39 ◆ CARE OF THE FAMILIES OF HIGH-RISK NEONATES

Page numbers in parentheses refer to textbook pages.

Clinical simulations

1. The Ayers are experiencing denial—one of the most common first reactions to the birth of a high-risk neonate. The perinatal team is concerned because although denial serves a protective purpose for a brief time, as long as the Ayers cling to denial they cannot participate in care decisions or make realistic plans. Should Ana die, they may be unable to grieve appropriately. (page 987)

2. To evaluate grieving behavior accurately, the nurse should consider cultural customs that may affect grief expression. However, assess carefully before drawing conclusions about a person's expression of grief: Although characteristic grieving behaviors typify certain cultures, these behaviors can change over time. Also, a person born into one culture but socialized in another may be influenced by elements of both.

   In the Ayers' case, keep in mind that Hispanic cultures typically regard public expression of grief as acceptable for the mother but not for the father, in whom they view it as a sign of weakness. (page 990)

3. The nurse asks the Ayers this question because incorporating health-related cultural or religious customs into Ana's care can help reduce their anxiety. Although nearly all parents feel intimidated during their first visit to the NICU, those who have deep religious beliefs or belong to an ethnic group with strong cultural identity and traditional health practices may feel particularly uncomfortable. Practices that pose no health threat or that can be modified so that they are safe can be incorporated fairly easily into Ana's care routine. If having such items as medallions, crosses, special clothes, prayer cards, or candles near Ana would comfort the Ayers, the nurse may place them near her, keeping safety foremost in mind. (page 993)

4. Interventions needed by family members immediately before and after a neonate's death depend partly on the relationship each has formed with the neonate and on the stage of grief each is in. To facilitate healthy grieving, the nurse should implement interventions that help Carmelita and Jorge complete their bonding with Ana as their child and a member of their family, building memories to sustain them in the future—a prerequisite to the eventual resolution of their grief.

   Also plan interventions to help the Ayers deal with their grief. Do not force them past denial, but provide and reinforce clear, accurate information about Ana's condition. Keep them informed of changes in her condition, and assure them that the staff will try to let them know when her death appears imminent so that they can be with her. (pages 998 and 999)

5. No. The nurse should not expect the Greenes to achieve complete resolution of their grief before Josie's discharge because this usually takes at least several months. Patrick's chronic disability may make complete acceptance difficult or even impossible to achieve. His chronic condition will necessitate continual adaptation and coping; the disability and the limitations it places on his life will remain a constant cause of sorrow for the Greenes. (page 987)

6. To enhance the Greenes' mutual support, the nurse should promote communication between them and provide opportunities for them to discuss their feelings. (page 994)

7. Unless Kevin's needs receive attention, he may face lifelong problems in dealing with the changes that the birth of a sibling such as Patrick creates. He may develop communication problems and may experience conflicting feelings about Patrick.

   Besides helping the Greenes balance Patrick's and Kevin's need for attention, the nurse should make sure they are aware of the feelings Kevin may be experiencing. For instance, he may sense their fear or worry over Patrick's chronic condition; he may feel guilty or be jealous or angry that Patrick takes up so much of their time and energy. Encourage the Greenes to spend time with Kevin and explain Patrick's condition in terms he can understand. Promote interaction between the brothers, and explore ways that other family members might help with housekeeping so that when Josie and Mike are home, they can devote attention and energy to family interaction, not just to Patrick's care. (pages 994 to 996)

8. The NICU nurse should be sensitive to the grandparents' needs because they share many of the parents' difficulties in coping with the neonate's condition and may feel an extra burden because of their role in the family. Also, nursing sensitivity to the unique needs of grandparents may enhance family-centered care after the birth of a preterm neonate. For instance, giving Margery's parents access to accurate information might relieve some of Margery's burden to provide information about her daughter's status. Opportunities for emotional support and education might help decrease the grandparents' anxiety and thus help them support Margery. This in turn would reaffirm their important role in the family. (pages 991 and 996)

Study questions

9. Kübler-Ross described five stages of grief: denial, anger, bargaining, depression, and acceptance. (page 986)

10. Bowlby, Parkes, and Davidson proposed four dimensions of grief that survivors of loss may move among: shock and numbness, yearning and searching, disorientation, and reorganization. (page 986)

11. Because the stages of grief are descriptive rather than clearly defined, parents and other family members may experience aspects of several stages at once or may regress to a stage previously experienced, instead of progressing through the stages in an orderly manner. (page 986)

12. Nursing assessment of the neonate's parents should include their age, experience as parents, and previous childbirth history; their understanding of and feelings about the neonate's condition; their concerns about the neonate's care; family and home care arrangements; their response to the NICU; and their grieving behaviors and coping mechanisms. (page 988)

13. For most parents, the first line of support comes from within the family; in a two-parent family, the partners typically form each other's base of support. Other potential sources of support include close friends, religious practices, cultural customs, and community support groups consisting of other parents in similar circumstances. (pages 989 and 990)

14. Four general nursing interventions for the family of a high-risk neonate are providing information, strengthening support systems, teaching caregiving skills, and enhancing parent-infant bonding. (page 992)

15. To determine whether parents need further nursing intervention before the neonate's discharge, the nurse should assess for such behaviors as a delay in arranging for medical support equipment in the home, infrequent calls or visits to the NICU, and apparent lack of interest in giving simple care to their child in the NICU. (page 998)

16. To involve the parents in the high-risk neonate's care, the nurse should increase the family's comfort level by arranging for the neonate and parents to be together as much as possible, let them participate in basic care as the neonate's condition permits, involve them in developmental care to reduce the physical and mental limitations of high-risk birth, and invite their participation in decision making about their child's daily care. (pages 996 and 997)

ANSWERS FOR CHAPTER 40 • DISCHARGE PLANNING AND NEONATAL CARE AT HOME

Page numbers in parentheses refer to textbook pages.

Clinical simulations

1. To determine the Harrises' discharge needs, the nurse should assess their ability and willingness to care for Scott at home, ability to bond with Scott, understanding of growth and development, knowledge of neonatal and infant care techniques, physical and psychosocial support systems, need for additional caregivers, stress level, medical insurance and financial resources, and psychosocial adaptation to the changing family structure. (pages 1009 and 1010)

2. To provide proper care for Scott, the Harrises must understand apnea and the purpose of the home apnea monitor, know the correct monitor settings and operation, understand safety precautions, know how to respond to monitor alarms, be able to keep an accurate apnea log, and be able to perform infant cardiopulmonary resuscitation. (page 1019)

3. The nurse should assess the parents' ability and willingness to care for Kevin at home, especially since his mother also has AIDS. Determine how much his parents know about the disease and the care Kevin will require. Also find out if they know the precautions necessary to prevent disease spread to other family members. (page 1025)

Study questions

4. Discharge planning should begin when the neonate is delivered or, at the latest, by nursery admission. The nurse continues to assess the neonate's and family's discharge planning needs until the neonate is discharged. (page 1031)

5. The nurse's major discharge planning responsibilities include developing a discharge plan, making referrals as necessary to help the family cope with the neonate's condition; integrating the neonate into the family; providing the family with health education to promote neonatal and infant care; and initiating and participating in neonatal care conferences with the family and other members of the health care team. (page 1008)

6. Typically, in-facility resource personnel involved in discharge planning include the clinical nurse specialist; physician; social worker; financial counselor; speech, hearing, occupational, and physical therapists; utilization review nurse; dietitian; respiratory therapist; and child life therapist. (page 1009)

7. Alternatives to home care for neonates and infants needing continued medical care include foster care, nursing homes, transitional infant care programs, and prescribed pediatric extended care facilities. (page 1012)

8. The nurse should teach the parents caregiving skills, emergency interventions, signs and symptoms of medical problems, use of special equipment, and names of people to contact when they have questions. Teaching strategies may incorporate verbal and written instruction, demonstration, and videotapes. (page 1031)

9. The nurse must make sure the medical record includes an assessment of the neonate's needs, problems, capabilities, and limitations; evidence of parental participation in discharge planning; evidence of parental learning of information provided; availability of recommended services for the family; the neonate's medical status at discharge; and the actual discharge plan, including prescribed medications, follow-up medical appointments, and any referrals to community agencies. (page 1014)

10. Case management is most helpful for parents who lack the ability or means to coordinate their child's care and for those whose child has multiple needs necessitating the involvement of several agencies and support services. (page 1016)

11. The ventilator-dependent neonate receiving care at home usually has a decreased infection risk, greater socialization, and better stimulation for growth and development. (page 1016)

12. Members of parent support groups have had firsthand experience in caring for special-needs children and can offer advice on which problems to anticipate, how to cope with problems, and where to find special supplies or services. (page 1021)

ANSWERS FOR CHAPTER 41 ◆ PHYSIOLOGY OF THE POSTPARTAL PERIOD

Page numbers in parentheses refer to textbook pages.

1. The nurse should inform Ms. Hannaberry that she is experiencing afterpains, strong myometrial contractions that resemble labor pains and shrink the uterus to the size of a grapefruit. Mention that many multiparous clients have more intense postpartal contractions than primiparous clients—probably because uterine muscles become less elastic with each pregnancy and must work harder to regain their shape. Inform her that lactation also promotes more severe contractions because oxytocin, the hormone that regulates milk ejection, stimulates uterine muscles. (page 1038)

2. The nurse should explain that lochia is considered abnormal if it contains large clots or tissue fragments (pieces of tissue, not the tissue debris normal to lochial flow), if it has a foul or offensive odor, or if its color or amount relapses to that of a previous stage. (page 1041)

3. The nurse-midwife should explain that the vaginal epithelium becomes fragile and atrophic by the third or fourth postpartal week because of the decreased estrogen level. In the nonlactating client, vaginal atrophy resolves by 6 to 10 weeks postpartum as estrogen normalizes. However, the breast-feeding client may continue to experience symptoms of atrophy, such as decreased vaginal lubrication and diminished sexual response, because the estrogen level remains low during lactation. (page 1041)

4. The nurse should inform Ms. Delaney and other class members that although lactation delays the return of a normal menstrual cycle, the length of the delay depends on breast-feeding duration and frequency. Thus, a client who breast-feeds exclusively for 6 months has longer-lasting amenorrhea than one who breast-feeds for 4 weeks. Likewise, the more regularly an infant breast-feeds without nutritional supplementation, the less likely that a woman will resume her menses because of natural hormonal suppression.

   Explain that the return of ovulation also varies. For both nonlactating and lactating women, an increased interval before the first postpartal menses increases the likelihood of an ovulatory cycle. Emphasize that because ovulation takes place 2 weeks before the start of menses, a woman who breast-feeds for several months may be fertile without advance warning. Consequently, caution breast-feeding clients not to rely on amenorrhea as contraception during the postpartal period. (pages 1043 and 1044)

5. The nurse should advise Ms. Saltz that she should not to expect to fit into her normal clothing for the first 6 to 8 postpartal weeks—until the structural changes of pregnancy have reversed. Inform her that enlargement of the breasts and abdominal wall muscles during pregnancy weakens these structures. Also mention that during the third trimester, fetal growth can cause separation of the rec-

tus abdominis muscles; this condition, which may persist indefinitely unless adequate muscle tone is restored, is exacerbated by the weight of the uterus, which remains somewhat enlarged. Mention that the pelvic joints, loosened by the abdominal distention caused by pregnancy, also remain relaxed. Reassure Ms. Saltz that these structural changes reverse gradually over the first 6 to 8 postpartal weeks. (page 1048)

6. The nurse should assess Ms. Yarrow's temperature to rule out fever or infection, then explain that many clients experience episodes of profuse diaphoresis (sweating) during the first 2 to 3 postpartal days. Associated with the postpartal fluid shift, diaphoresis is a normal mechanism that helps the renal system excrete excess fluid and waste products. Reassure Ms. Yarrow that the problem should resolve within 1 week. (pages 1048 and 1049)

7. The nurse should expect to palpate Ms. Beyer's uterus one fingerbreadth below the umbilicus. (pages 1038 and 1039)

Study questions

8. The myometrium (uterine muscle) and endometrium (uterine lining) help the uterus return to nonpregnant state. (page 1037)

9. The uterine mechanisms that cause uterine involution are myometrial contractions and autolysis. Myometrial contractions beginning immediately after delivery of the placenta shrink the uterus to roughly half its immediate predelivery size. This forces the uterine walls into close proximity, causing the center cavity to flatten. Through autolysis—self-disintegration or self-digestion—hypertrophic uterine cells return to a nonpregnant shape and size. The byproducts of autolyzed cellular protein are absorbed and excreted by the renal system. (pages 1037, 1038, and 1040)

10. The uterus regains a nonpregnant weight and size within 6 weeks. (page 1038)

11. Lochia is the vaginal discharge that appears during the postpartal period. It has three distinct stages. The first stage, lochia rubra, typically lasts 3 to 4 days. It is bright red; contains a mixture of mucus, tissue debris, and blood; and has a slightly fleshy odor. The second stage, lochia serosa, occurs as uterine bleeding subsides. Lochia serosa is more serous than lochia rubra, appearing pink or brownish. Usually odorless, it persists for 5 to 7 days postpartum. Lochia alba, the third stage, is a creamy white, brown, or colorless discharge consisting mainly of serum and white blood cells. It usually subsides after 3 weeks, but may persist for 6 weeks or longer. It may have a slightly stale odor. (pages 1040 and 1041)

12. Resumption of the menstrual cycle is coordinated by interaction of the hypothalamus, which produces gonadotropin-releasing hormone; the pituitary gland, which secretes follicle-stimulating hormone and luteinizing hormone; and the ovaries, which produce estrogen and progesterone. (page 1043)

13. The mechanisms that help restore normal blood volume after delivery are blood loss during delivery, extravascular fluid shift, a decrease in the vascular bed, and hormonal influence. Blood loss after delivery reduces blood volume immediately. (The pregnancy-related increase in blood volume allows the body to withstand substantial blood loss during delivery.) The postpartal shift of extravascular fluid to the circulation leads to a plasma volume increase that helps offset blood loss at delivery. (This fluid is excreted as postpartal diuresis occurs.) After delivery of the placenta, the vascular bed shrinks considerably; thus, a smaller blood volume is needed for tissue perfusion. The vasodilatory effects of hormonal tissue disappear after delivery, reducing the amount of blood required to maintain adequate tissue perfusion and blood pressure. (page 1045)

14. The nurse should discuss the danger signs of thrombophlebitis because postpartal clients are at risk for thromboembolic disorders. Throughout pregnancy, levels of coagulation factors VII, IX, X and fibrinogen rise progressively; during late pregnancy, fibrinolysis diminishes. Thus the pregnant client has a progressively increasing risk for thromboembolic disorders. Delivery stimulates the coagulation system, increasing this risk even further in the early postpartal period. Coagulation factors remain significantly elevated for the first 2 to 3 weeks postpartum. (page 1046)

15. Postpartally, abdominal muscle tone may be so poor that the client cannot attain sufficient pressure to evacuate the bowel. Also, the client may avoid bowel evacuation, fearing it will cause pain or damage the episiotomy. Residual dehydration from labor and the subsequent decrease in fluid content of the stool also may impair bowel evacuation. (page 1047)

16. *Uterus.* Enlarged greatly during pregnancy, the uterus shrinks dramatically during the early postpartal period. However, it never resumes its nulliparous size and shape. (P) (page 1038)
Cervix. After dilating during labor and delivery, the cervix resumes its normal functional anatomy. After vaginal delivery, it never regains its nulliparous appearance. (P) (page 1041)
Breasts. Within 3 months after delivery, connective and adipose tissue replace the glandular breast tissue that increased during pregnancy. The breasts typically resume nonpregnancy size; however, a mild alteration in breast shape may be permanent. (P) (page 1043)
Respiratory system. After delivery, pregnancy-related respiratory changes and associated complaints (such as shortness of breath, chest and rib discomfort, and decreased tolerance for physical exertion) resolve completely. (T) (page 1044)
Cardiovascular system. Cardiac enlargement and displacement, caused by the enlarged pregnant uterus, reverse after delivery as the uterus resumes its normal size and shape. (T) (page 1044)
Immune system. Inhibited during pregnancy to prevent rejection of the fetus as foreign matter, the immune system resumes normal functioning after delivery. (T) (page 1049)

Skin. Striae (stretch marks) occur during pregnancy from increased corticosteroid levels and mechanical stretching of the skin. They shrink and fade within 1 year after delivery but never disappear completely. (P) (page 1048)

Metabolic system. Throughout pregnancy, the basal metabolic rate rises. It decreases rapidly to a nonpregnancy level, approaching nonpregnancy levels by 5 to 6 days postpartum. (T) (page 1049)

Page numbers in parentheses refer to textbook pages.

Clinical simulations

1. Because Ms. Aguirre lacks other signs of infection, the nurse should suspect that her slight temperature elevation stems from mild dehydration caused by labor and delivery. This condition—common during the first 24 hours postpartum—is clinically insignificant. (page 1052)

2. The nurse should keep in mind that Ms. Aguirre did not lose excessive blood during delivery, her blood pressure and respiratory rate are normal, and she is not pale or diaphoretic. Therefore, interpret her increased pulse rate as a reflection of her excitement and afterbirth pains rather than a dangerous condition, such as shock. (page 1052)

3. To reduce Ms. Aguirre's discomfort from afterbirth pains, the nurse should assist her to the bathroom to void (afterbirth pains may stem from a full bladder). As prescribed, offer her an analgesic or a nonsteroidal anti-inflammatory drug. (pages 1059 and 1061)

4. The nurse should recognize that a persistent blood pressure elevation signals pregnancy-induced hypertension (PIH)—especially when accompanied by such signs and symptoms as headache, visual changes, and edema. Check for proteinuria and hyperactive reflexes—other signs of PIH—and review Ms. Neborsky's antepartal and intrapartal records for a history of PIH. To ensure prompt intervention, report Ms. Neborsky's signs and symptoms to the physician immediately. (page 1053)

5. A soft, boggy uterus reflects uterine atony (poor muscle tone). This condition, which may lead to hemorrhage, typically stems from bladder distention or uterine enlargement. Because of Ms. Jordan's multiparity and her neonate's large size, the nurse should suspect uterine enlargement as the cause of atony in this case. Such enlargement results in overstretching of muscle fibers, which then cannot contract effectively to compress uterine vessels. An accelerated labor also can lead to uterine atony by exhausting uterine muscles. (page 1053)

6. The nurse should attempt to have Ms. Kohan void spontaneously because postpartal bladder distention can lead to uterine atony. To promote spontaneous voiding, encourage Ms. Kohan to walk to the bathroom; if she is confined to bed, offer her a bedpan. Other nursing interventions that promote spontaneous voiding include turning on the bathroom faucet, irrigating the perineum, place the client's hands in water, and providing plenty of fluids. (pages 1053 and 1059)

7. The combination of excessive blood loss at delivery, elevated pulse and respiratory rates, decreased blood pressure, and lochia flowing in a steady trickle suggests that Ms. Jenkins is experiencing postpartal hemorrhage. The consistency and location of the fundus and lochial characteristics suggest cervical or vaginal laceration as the most likely cause of hemorrhage. (pages 1052 and 1056)

8. To reduce Ms. Farrell's episiotomy pain, the nurse should apply an ice pack to the perineum, which soothes the area by constricting vessels and reducing the vascular response of inflammation. The nurse can use a commercial perineal ice pack or make one by filling a latex glove with ice and knotting it at the top.

   To promote perineal healing, provide for application of warmth to the perineum, such as with sitz baths, as prescribed. Other comfort measures include application of a topical spray, topical ointment, or witch hazel compresses; a commercial water and disinfectant spray; perineal heat lamp treatments, and mild analgesics. To promote perineal hygiene, instruct Ms. Farrell to perform perineal irrigation after voiding or moving her bowels. (pages 1062 and 1063)

9. The nurse should suspect that Mrs. Cheng has postspinal headache, which may result from loss of cerebrospinal fluid through the dural puncture site. Position Mrs. Cheng flat; if she is permitted to lie on her side, make sure her head is elevated no more than 30 degrees. Ensure that she remains supine for 8 to 10 hours after anesthesia administration. Monitor her response to positioning; if she reports that the headache has worsened, lower the head of the bed. Be sure to notify the physician of her condition promptly. (pages 1057 and 1064)

Multiple choice

10. (b) (page 1053)

11. (c). This finding usually signifies breast engorgement, a common discomfort of the early postpartal period. (page 1054)

Study questions

12. Signs of postpartal hemorrhage include a boggy uterus; an excessively large uterus located above the umbilicus at the midline; excessive lochia, possibly containing large blood clots with or without tissue fragments, lochia that flows in a steady trickle; and increased pulse and respiratory rates with decreased blood pressure. (page 1056)

13. The episiotomy should appear to be healing with no exudate; the site should be clean and not excessively tender; and such abnormalities as redness, warmth, tenderness, edema, ecchymosis, and discharge should be absent. (page 1054)

14. Urinary catheterization is necessary because bladder distention can prevent uterine contractions and vessel compression, causing excessive uterine bleeding. (pages 1056 and 1059)

15. The nurse must evaluate the lower extremities carefully because the postpartal client is predisposed to thromboembolic disease, a condition that results from hypercoagulability caused by decreased

plasma volume. To assess for thromboembolic disease, have the client lie supine with both legs extended. Inspect the legs for symmetry of shape and size and palpate the thighs and calves to detect areas of warmth, edema, tenderness, redness, and hardness. Then attempt to elicit Homan's sign. (page 1057)

16. Such factors as blood loss, fatigue, limited food intake, and medication effects may contribute to weakness and light-headedness for the first few hours after delivery; injury may result. To ensure safety, the nurse should instruct the client to call for help when getting out of bed for the first time and show her how to raise or lower the bed rails. To prevent injury to the neonate, caution the client against falling asleep in bed with the neonate. (page 1059)

17. The nurse should teach the client to avoid stimulation of the breasts (such as from a shower stream flowing directly onto the breasts and nipples) and to wear a tight support bra or breast binder. Inform her that she may notice an occasional release of milk and may experience breast fullness and discomfort until milk production ceases. Encourage her to drink adequate but not excessive amounts of fluids. Recommend a mild analgesic or application of ice packs for severe breast discomfort. Also teach her about signs of breast infection. (pages 1063, 1067, and 1068)

18. To increase comfort for the client with hemorrhoids, the nurse can apply witch hazel compresses soaked in ice chips, use an anesthetic or steroid-based cream, administer antihemorrhoidal suppositories or mild analgesics, encourage sitz baths, and position the client on her side. (page 1064)

19. The Rh-negative client who delivers an Rh-positive neonate should receive Rh immune globulin (RhoGAM) to prevent isoimmunization. The injection should be given within 72 hours of delivery. (page 1064)

20. Multiparous postpartal clients have more affective than psychomotor concerns. Therefore, the nurse should center teaching around such topics as how to meet the needs of other children, find time for themselves, and regain a positive body image while caring for their neonate. (page 1067)

21. Respiratory assessment is especially crucial for this client because surgical delivery increases the risk of respiratory complications. To check for altered breathing patterns and poor gas exchange, auscultate the client's lungs every 4 hours for adventitious sounds, such as crackles or rhonchi. Evaluate the breathing pattern regularly until the lungs are free of adventitious sounds and the client is ambulatory. (page 1056)

ANSWERS FOR CHAPTER 43 • PSYCHOSOCIAL ADAPTATION OF THE POSTPARTAL FAMILY

Page numbers in parentheses refer to textbook pages.

Clinical simulations

1. Ms. Styler's poor eye contact with Abby, avoidance of close physical contact with her, and harsh vocal tone suggest poor maternal attachment. Potential consequences of poor attachment include vulnerable child syndrome, child abuse, failure to thrive, and a disturbed parent-child relationship. (pages 1076, 1082, and 1084)

2. A home visit would provide a good opportunity for Martha to observe Ms. Styler and Abby together in their own environment. If possible, Martha should observe them during a feeding session, when they are most likely to interact. To help ensure an accurate assessment, Martha should observe on at least two occasions; if Ms. Styler is fatigued or in discomfort during one observation, her behavior may give Martha a false impression. (page 1082)

3. Martha should assess Mr. Rausch's adaptation because this will help ensure family-centered care. Because of his role as Ms. Styler's main support person, his emotional status and adaptation to parenthood are especially important. To assess Mr. Rausch, Martha should stay alert for signs that he wants to unburden himself by talking about the childbirth experience and his feelings, determine his level of knowledge about neonatal behavior and care, and evaluate his expectations of Ms. Styler's postpartal recovery and his understanding of the time and energy involved in caring for a neonate. Martha also should check for signs that Mr. Rausch is disappointed that Ms. Styler did not have a son. (pages 1086 and 1087)

4. Martha's documentation of this visit should include signs or lack of signs of positive bonding, the quality of Ms. Styler's and Mr. Rausch's interaction with Abby, their ability to interpret and respond appropriately to Abby's communication cues, evidence of reciprocity and synchrony when Abby and her arents communicate, evidence of Ms. Styler's progression through the stages of maternal adaptation, Ms. Styler's emotional status, Mr. Rausch's emotional status and adaptation to parenthood, Ms. Styler's caregiving skills, and the adaptation of Ms. Styler's other children to Abby's birth. (page 1091)

5. Yes; all of the preconditions identified by Mercer are present. These preconditions include Ms. Robertson's apparent emotional health, her adequate social network (which includes both her and her husband's families), her competence in parental communication and caregiving skills, her access to her son, and her temperamental compatibility with her neonate. (page 1076)

6. Ms. Ritsick's age affects her capacity for bonding with her neonate as well as her readiness to assume the maternal role. Her response

is typical of an adolescent mother, who usually lacks an established identity and a secure relationship with the neonate's father. Faced with parenting tasks and responsibilities as well as the typical adolescent concerns of school and social life, she may feel overwhelmed and resentful of the neonate. Also, she has her own dependency needs and probably is not mature enough to assume a full maternal role or meet her child's financial needs. Her support system may be inadequate and her friends and family may not be ready to accept her as a parent. (page 1080)

7. The nurse should expect Ms. Ritsick to have a greater need for teaching about neonatal and infant care. Because Ms. Ritsick lacks caregiving experience, be especially supportive; the seeming ease with which the nurse performs neonatal care may reinforce Ms. Ritsick's feelings of inadequacy. Supervise her as she cares for her neonate, offering praise and encouragement. Express confidence in her ability to cope with new tasks. (page 1088)

8. The nurse can begin by explaining that many siblings feel uncertain or jealous when a brother or sister is born. To help their daughters adjust, encourage the Mullers to have them visit their new brother in the health care facility before Ms. Muller's discharge. Urge Ms. Muller to call them on the telephone frequently and spend uninterrupted time with them when they visit. Instruct her and Tom to watch for both overt and covert signs of jealousy in the girls after they take their son home. (pages 1088 and 1089)

9. The four other essential parenting tasks that Ms. Samuels should include are psychological tasks, such as reconciling the real child with the fantasy child; gaining competence in caregiving skills; becoming sensitive to neonatal communication cues; and establishing the neonate's place within the family. (page 1075)

Study questions

10. The parent-child relationship sets the foundation for all other relationships the child will develop. The basic trust between parent and child that develops during infancy is crucial to the child's ability to form successful relationships. (page 1075)

11. The nurse can arrange for the parents to interact with the neonate immediately after a normal labor and delivery to take advantage of enhanced neonatal receptivity at this time. Urge them to get acquainted with the neonate by cuddling, touching, and exploring the neonate's body. If appropriate, encourage the client to initiate breast-feeding at this time. (page 1087)

12. Nurturing is an example of a cognitive- affective parenting skill—one that links mental processes with feelings or emotions. Diapering a neonate is an example of a cognitive-motor parenting skill—one that links mental processes with physical activities.
The nurse is more likely to incorporate cognitive- motor skills into parent teaching because such skills involve physical caregiving tasks and can be learned. In contrast, the emotional responses associated with cognitive-affective skills, are imprinted before the neonate's birth. (page 1075)

13. Assessment tools used to evaluate maternal adaptation include the neonatal perception inventory developed by Broussard, the maternal-infant observation scale created by Avant, and the Brazelton neonatal behavioral assessment scale. (page 1082)

Fill in the blank

14. acquaintance (page 1076)
15. boredom; overstimulation (page 1078)
16. reciprocity (page 1078)
17. synchrony (page 1078)
18. entrainment (page 1078)

True or false

19. False (page 1081)
20. False (page 1081)
21. True (page 1076)
22. True (page 1076)
23. False (pages 1080 and 1092)
24. True (page 1092)
25. True (page 1077)
26. True (page 1076)

Matching terms and definitions

27. (1) c, e, h; (2) f, g; (3) a, b, d (pages 1078 and 1080)

ANSWERS FOR CHAPTER 44 • POSTPARTAL COMPLICATIONS

Page numbers in parentheses refer to textbook pages.

Clinical simulations

1. The nurse should suspect puerperal infection. Signs and symptoms suggesting puerperal infection include chills, headache, a morbid temperature, a tender uterus, an increase in lochial flow, and foul-smelling lochia. (pages 1102 and 1103)

2. Many factors described in Ms. Fouillard's medical records increase the risk of puerperal infection. Her antepartal risk factors include anemia and poor nutrition; intrapartal risk factors include prolonged rupture of the membranes, intrauterine monitoring, numerous vaginal examinations, a prolonged labor, and cesarean delivery. (pages 1095, 1097, 1102, and 1103)

3. The nurse should expect the physician to order a complete blood count and an erythrocyte sedimentation rate. Be prepared to assist with collection of blood and vaginal cultures to identify the infecting organism. (page 1102)

4. Besides administering prescribed antimicrobial and antipyretic therapy, the nurse should implement measures that alleviate signs and symptoms of infection and meet Ms. Fouillard's psychosocial needs. Provide comfort measures, such as by administering a prescribed analgesic to relieve her headache; promote adequate rest; provide a relaxed, quiet environment to counter malaise; and ensure a fluid intake of 2,000 ml/day. Also teach her and her family about her condition and treatment, and provide emotional support and encouragement. Reassure her that her neonate is being cared for, and help her work through anxiety and discouragement by urging her to express her feelings. (page 1108)

5. Ms. Johnson's risk factors for thrombophlebitis include her age (over 40), obesity, parity greater than three, anemia, and previous history of venous thrombosis. (pages 1106 and 1111)

6. Pulmonary embolism is a possible complication of thrombophlebitis. To prevent pulmonary embolism, the nurse should implement such measures as local heat application, elevation of the affected limb, bed rest, analgesics, and use of elastic stockings to help prevent blood from pooling in the legs. Caution Ms. Johnson not to massage or rub the affected extremity. Once Ms. Johnson's symptoms subside, urge her to resume ambulation gradually. Instruct her to wear elastic support stockings and to perform prescribed leg exercises. Advise her not to stand or sit for long periods and to avoid crossing her legs because this reduces circulation. Teach her how to identify signs and symptoms of thrombus formation, and advise her to call the physician if they occur. Instruct her to manage symptoms and relieve pain by applying warm, moist soaks and taking analgesics. Throughout her stay in the postpartal unit, encourage fre-

quent visits with her daughter to promote mother-infant bonding. (paged 1106 and 1111)

7. The nurse should instruct Ms. Nathan to breast-feed her neonate every 2 to 3 hours, beginning on the affected side and continuing until the breast feels completely soft. Advise her to apply a warm, wet washcloth to the affected area immediately before feeding. Instruct her to breast-feed in different positions during each feeding session to promote full drainage of all milk ducts. Encourage her to massage the affected area gently while breast-feeding and to express or pump any remaining milk from the breast after breast-feeding.

   Discourage the use of a bra or other restrictive clothing when breast-feeding. Advise Ms. Nathan to increase her fluid take by several glasses, rest as much as possible, and ask family members or friends to help with child care and household chores. Instruct her to contact the physician if her neonate develops diarrhea or if she does not feel better after 48 hours of antibiotics and breast-feeding. (page 1112)

8. A substance-abusing postpartal client such as Ms. Ford will require a multidisciplinary treatment approach. Besides the nurse and physician, a social worker, child protection worker, and community health worker may be involved in her care. Treatment will depend on her willingness to admit her problem and comply with a drug treatment program.

   Besides routine documentation, the nurse must include the following items when documenting Ms. Ford's care:
   - signs and symptoms of drug withdrawal or continued drug use during hospitalization
   - response to prescribed analgesics
   - extent of her interaction with her neonate, partner, and the health care team
   - absence or presence of signs of mother-infant bonding
   - expressions of willingness to be treated for substance abuse. (pages 1113 and 1116)

9. Any condition causing trauma during childbirth can lead to postpartal hemorrhage. The nurse should consider retained placental fragments and lacerations of the vagina, cervix, perineum, or labia as possible causes of Ms. Greer's hemorrhage. (page 1098)

10. The nurse should inform Ms. Greer that a precipitous labor can cause a deep cervical laceration; such an injury can lead to serious hemorrhage because of the increased vascularity of the cervix and fragility of surrounding tissues. (page 1100)

11. Ms. Lincoln's history and clinical condition suggest a urinary tract disorder, such as cystitis or pyelonephritis. (page 1106)

12. The nurse should make sure Ms. LaRue understands the expected postpartal changes in her dietary and insulin requirements. Emphasize that she should remain flexible and patient because postpartal diabetes control may be difficult to achieve, causing frustration and

anger. Stress that she should not consider herself "cured" of diabetes if she can go 1 or 2 days without insulin and eat a regular diet during the postpartal period.

Inform Ms. Lincoln that she can breast-feed her neonate safely because insulin does not enter the breast milk. However, instruct her to consume an additional 300 to 500 calories daily to maintain breast-feeding; this will necessitate insulin adjustments, as may her altered postpartal sleeping and eating patterns. (pages 1112 and 1113)

Study questions

13. Predisposing factors for postpartal hemorrhage include cesarean delivery, delivery of a large neonate, forceps or mid forceps rotation at delivery, hematoma, hydramnios, intrauterine manipulation, lacerations of the birth canal, magnesium sulfate use during labor, manual removal of the placenta, multiparity, more than one fetus, premature placental separation, previous postpartal hemorrhage, prolonged labor, retained placental fragments, uterine atony, and uterine inversion. (page 1104)

14. The REEDA scale evaluates five components of perineal healing after an episiotomy or perineal laceration, providing a means for objective assessment. To use this scale, the nurse observes for redness, edema, ecchymosis, discharge, and approximation of the perineum. The total score may range from 1 to 15; the higher the total, the worse the condition of the perineum. (page 1105)

15. Infection-prevention measures include careful aseptic technique (especially thorough hand washing) and avoidance of cross-contamination among clients (for instance, by ensuring that each client has her own sanitary supplies and that nondisposable items are cleaned after each use). (pages 1107 and 1108)

16. The main goals of nursing care for the postpartal client with preeclampsia are prevention of seizures and close monitoring for signs and symptoms of the disorder. The ultimate goal is to stabilize the client's status by intervening appropriately, providing optimal environmental conditions, and promoting psychosocial adjustment. (page 1110)

17. Substance abuse may go undetected until the postpartal period because many pregnant substance abusers do not seek prenatal care. Even when signs of substance abuse manifest earlier, the client may deny her problem because of fear of the legal and social ramifications. (page 1102)

18. The nurse should instruct the family to observe the client for a depressed mood, markedly diminished interest or pleasure in activities, significant weight loss or gain, insomnia or hypersomnia, psychomotor agitation, fatigue, feelings of worthlessness, excessive or inappropriate guilt, diminished ability to think, and recurrent thoughts of death. Mention that the client also may show a lack of bonding with her neonate or may express overt hostility and a desire to harm herself. She may feel unable to love her neonate and may lose the ability to cope with family life and its everyday tasks.

Inform the family that supportive therapy, such as psychiatric consultation, should begin as early as possible if signs or symptoms appear. (pages 1107 and 1113)

Fill in the blank

19. a morbid temperature (pages 1102 and 1117)

20. identifying its cause (page 1117)

21. Kegel exercises (page 1117)

22. fluctuate widely (page 1112)

23. rectum; vagina (page 1100)

ANSWERS FOR CHAPTER 45 • MATERNAL CARE AT HOME

Page numbers in parentheses refer to textbook pages.

Clinical simulations

1. The nurse should determine if the home is conducive to safe, adequate care of Ms. Brown and her neonate and whether it promotes positive psychosocial adaptation. Check for safety hazards and the availability of basic necessities, such as water, electricity, and heat. Also determine whether Ivy can obtain privacy in the home. (page 1124)

2. To evaluate Ms. Brown's psychosocial status and adaptation to the maternal role more fully, the nurse should explore her feelings about the childbirth experience and assess her self-esteem. To adapt to her new role, Ms. Brown must relive and understand the events of childbirth so that she can incorporate them into her life and self-concept. Ask her what thoughts and feelings she has when looking back at the experience, how she thinks she handled the experience, and what aspects of the experience stand out in her mind. To evaluate her self-esteem, ask her how she would rate herself now in terms of goodness, how well she feels she is adjusting, what thoughts and feelings she has had about her physical attractiveness since the delivery, what her predominant mood is, and how she views her future. (page 1122)

3. To enhance Ms. Brown and Mr. Michelson's competence and confidence in parenting and caring for their neonate, the nurse should reinforce discharge teaching of neonatal caregiving skills and provide information about infant growth and development. Consider recommending fourth trimester classes, which provide anticipatory guidance and serve as a forum for parents to share their concerns. Also teach them about their neonate's capacities and behavioral traits. (page 1127)

4. To determine the severity of Ms. Edelson's mood swings, the nurse should note the onset, duration, and nature of her symptoms. Postpartal mood swings may take the form of "maternity blues," a more severe mood alteration, or a major depressive episode.
"Maternity blues" typically arises during the first 3 postpartal weeks; lasts approximately 1 to 10 days; and is characterized by sadness, crying episodes, fatigue, and low self-esteem. A more severe mood alteration usually arises within a few weeks of delivery and may last from several weeks to a year or more; the client becomes tearful, despondent, and guilt-ridden, with feelings of inadequacy and inability to cope with neonatal care. A major depressive episode, a rare condition, manifests as five or more of the following symptoms: depressed mood, markedly diminished interest or pleasure in activities, pronounced weight loss or gain, insomnia or hypersomnia, psychomotor agitation, fatigue or energy loss, feelings of worthlessness, diminished ability to think, and recurrent thoughts of death. The onset, duration, and nature of Ms. Edelson's

symptoms suggest that she has a more serious mood alteration than "maternity blues" but is not experiencing a major depressive episode. (pages 1123 and 1124)

Multiple choice

5. (d). A spontaneous visit is undesirable because the client may be away, entertaining visitors, or caring for older children when the nurse drops by. Setting specific appointment times helps minimize the likelihood of poor timing. (pages 1120 and 1121)

6. (b). The institutional setting legitimizes and formalizes the caregiver's role. In the home and other noninstitutional settings, the client might perceive certain nursing procedures as an invasion of privacy. (pages 1119 and 1121)

Study questions

7. The basic elements of this assessment include the history, physical examination, psychosocial assessment, evaluation of mother-infant interaction, and evaluation of the home. (page 1121)

8. For the client receiving care at home, major nursing goals include promoting postpartal recovery, helping the client adapt to the maternal role, promoting parenting skills, enhancing the couple's relationship, and helping siblings adapt to the birth of a new family member. (page 1125)

9. The nurse should note whether the pregnancy was planned or unplanned; the extent of the client's prenatal care; exposures during pregnancy (such as smoking, alcohol, or drugs); and hospital admissions or problems during pregnancy. (page 1122)

True or false

10. False (page 1125)

11. False (page 1125)

12. True (page 1125)

13. False (page 1121)

14. True (page 1129)

15. False (page 1125)

Matching exercise

16. (1) b, f; (2) d, i; (3) a, g; (4) c, e, h (page 1128)